The International Library of Psychology

THE ELEMENTS OF PSYCHOLOGY

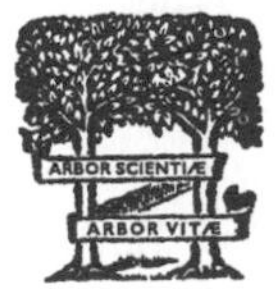

Founded by C. K. Ogden

The International Library of Psychology

GENERAL PSYCHOLOGY
In 38 Volumes

I	The Neurosis of Man	*Burrow*
II	Creative Imagination	*Downey*
III	The Caveman Within Us	*Fielding*
IV	Men and their Motives	*Flugel*
V	The Mind in Sleep	*Fortune*
VI	The Mind and its Body	*Fox*
VII	Practical Psychology	*Fox*
VIII	Man for Himself	*Fromm*
IX	The Law Within	*Fuller*
X	The Nature of Laughter	*Gregory*
XI	Readings in General Psychology	*Halmos et al*
XII	The Psychologist at Work	*Harrower*
XIII	The Psychology of Philosophers	*Herzberg*
XIV	Emotion	*Hillman*
XV	The Foundations of Common Sense	*Isaacs*
XVI	The Psychology of Consciousness	*King*
XVII	The Sciences of Man in the Making	*Kirkpatrick*
XVIII	The Person in Psychology	*Lafitte*
XIX	Man's Unconscious Passion	*Lay*
XX	Psychological and Biological Foundations of Dream-Interpretation	*Lowy*
XXI	Nervous Disorders and Character	*Mckenzie*
XXII	An Historical Introduction to Modern Psychology	*Murphy*
XXIII	Modern Theories of the Unconscious	*Northridge*
XXIV	The A B C of Psychology	*Ogden*
XXV	The Psychology of Thought and Feeling	*Platt*
XXVI	Introductory Psychology	*Price-Williams*
XXVII	Empirical Foundations of Psychology	*Pronko et al*
XXVIII	Psychotherapy	*Schilder*
XXIX	The Psychology of Time	*Sturt*
XXX	The Origins of Love and Hate	*Suttie*
XXXI	Art and the Unconscious	*Thorburn*
XXXII	The Elements of Psychology	*Thorndike*
XXXIII	Telepathy and Clairvoyance	*Tischner*
XXXIV	Human Psychology as Seen Through the Dream	*Turner*
XXXV	The Psychology of Self-Conciousness	*Turner*
XXXVI	The Psychology of Economics	*Weisskopf*
XXXVII	The Measurement of Emotion	*Whately Smith*
XXXVIII	How to be Happy Though Human	*Wolfe*

THE ELEMENTS OF PSYCHOLOGY

EDWARD L THORNDIKE

Introduction by William James

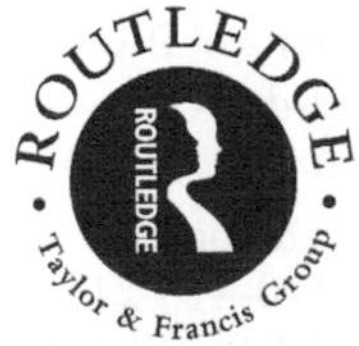

First published in 1905 by
Routledge

Reprinted in 1999, 2001 by
Routledge

2 Park Square, Milton Park, Abingdon, Oxfordshire OX14 4RN

711 Third Avenue, New York, NY 10017

Transferred to Digital Printing 2007

First issued in paperback 2014

Routledge is an imprint of the Taylor and Francis Group, an informa company

British Library Cataloguing in Publication Data
A CIP catalogue record for this book
is available from the British Library

The Elements of Psychology
ISBN 978-0-415-21044-7 (hbk)
ISBN 978-0-415-75809-3 (pbk)

General Psychology: 38 Volumes
ISBN 978-0-415-21129-1
The International Library of Psychology: 204 Volumes
ISBN 978-0-415-19132-6

INTRODUCTION

I have been invited to contribute a preface to this book, though when I ask myself, why any book from Professor Thorndike's pen should need an introduction to the public by another hand, I find no answer. Both as an experimental investigator, as a critic of other investigators, and as an expounder of results, he stands in the very forefront of American psychologists, and his references to my works in the text that follows will, I am sure, introduce me to more readers than I can introduce him to by my preface.

In addition to the monographs which have been pouring from the press for twenty years past, we have by this time, both in English and in German, a very large number of general text-books, some larger and some smaller, but all covering the ground in ways which, so far as students go, are practical equivalents for each other. The main subdivisions, principles, and features of descriptive psychology are at present well made out, and writers are agreed about them. If one has read earlier books, one need not read the very newest one in order to catch up with the progress of the science. The differences in them are largely of order and emphasis, or of fondness on the authors' parts for certain phrases, or for their own modes of approach to particular questions. It is one and the same body of facts with which they all make us acquainted.

Some of these treatises indeed give much more prominence to the details of experimentation than others—

artificial experimentation, I mean, with physical instruments, and measurements. A rapid glance at Professor Thorndike's table of contents might lead one to set him down as not belonging to the experimental class of psychologists. He ignores the various methods of proving Fechner's psycho-physic law, and makes no reference to chronoscopes, or to acoustical or optical technics. Yet in another and psychologically in a more vital sense his book is a laboratory manual of the most energetic and continuous kind.

When I first looked at the proofs and saw each section followed by a set of neatly numbered exercises, problems, and questions in fine print, I confess that I shuddered for a moment. Can it be, I thought, that the author's long connection with the Teachers College is making even of him a high-priest of the American "text-book" Moloch, in whose belly living children's minds are turned to ashes, and whose ritual lies in text-books in which the science is pre-digested for the teacher by every expository artifice and for the pupil comminuted into small print and large print, and paragraph-headings, and cross-references and examination questions, and every other up-to-date device for frustrating the natural movement of the mind when reading, and preventing that irresponsible rumination of the material in one's own way which is the soul of culture? Can it be, I said, that Thorndike himself is sacrificing to machinery and discontinuity?

But I had not read many of the galleys before I got the opposite impression. There are, it is true, discontinuities in the book which might slightly disconcert a critic with a French turn of taste, but that is because of the intense concreteness with which the author feels his subject and wishes to make his reader feel it. The problems and questions are uniquely to that end. They are laboratory work of the most continuous description, and the text is like unto them for concreteness. Professor Thorndike has more horror of vagueness, of scholastic phrases, of scientific humbug than any psychologist with whom I am acquainted. I defy any teacher or student to go through this book as it is written, and not to carry away an absolutely first-hand acquaintance with the workings of the human mind, and with the realities as distinguished from the pedantries and artificialities of psychology. The author's superabounding fertility in familiar illustrations of what he is describing amounts to genius. I might enter into an exposition of some of the other peculiarities of his treatise, but this quality of exceeding realism seems to cap the others and to give it eminence among the long list of psychology-books which readers now-a-days have to choose from.

It is not a work for lazy readers, however; and lazy reading also has a sacred place in the universe of education. But I seem to foresee for it a powerful anti-pedantic influence, and I augur for it a very great success indeed in class-rooms. So, with no more prefatory words, I heartily recommend it to all those who are interested in spreading the knowledge of our science.

William James.

Harvard University.

PREFACE

The aim of this book is to help students to learn the general principles of psychology. Those facts which can most profitably be made the subject matter of a course in general psychology are presented with an abundance of concrete illustrations, experiments, exercises and questions, by which the student may secure real rather than verbal conceptions and may test, apply and make permanent his knowledge.

A good method of studying the book is probably (1) to read a section through quickly, then (2) to read it with care, jotting down in a note book every *question* that seems to be answered by the text. Next (3) without the book try to answer those questions; hunting out the answers when unable to give them from memory. (4) Do the printed exercises, writing down each answer or, if it is too long, its main point. (5) Do any experiments in connection with the section. (6) When the several sections of a chapter have all been thus studied, write down the general questions which the whole chapter has answered, and after an interval of several days try to give clear and reasonably adequate answers to these questions in writing.

The references for further reading noted at the end of each chapter may best be read only after the text itself is mastered. The references marked A are for students in general, those marked B are for students especially desirous of increasing their knowledge of psychology and capable of studying difficult treatises. Additional readings on special topics will be found at the end of the book. In the references Roman numerals refer to the chapters. § 1, § 2, § 3, etc., refer to sections. Arabic numerals alone refer to pages. 'Titchener, *Outline*' refers to the third edition, that of 1899; 'Wundt, *Physiologische Psychologie*,' refers to the fifth edition.

The references to Wundt through Chapter VI are available in the English translation by Professor Titchener (*Principles of Physiological Psychology*, Vol. 1). Further volumes of this English version will appear in the near future.

Through the great kindness of Professor L. F. Barker of Chicago University, Professor Dr. L. Edinger of Frankfurt-a.M., Professor A. von Kölliker of Würzburg, Professor M. v. Lenhossék of Budapest, Professor M. Allen Starr, Dr. E. Leaming and Dr. O. S. Strong of Columbia University, and Professor A. Van Gehuchten of Louvain, I am able to reproduce photographs and drawings of the finer structure of the nervous system such as are rarely seen in elementary books on either psychology or physiology.

To Professor William James I owe the common debt of all psychologists due for the genius which has been our inspiration and the scholarship which has been our guide. The obligation is patent in every chapter. Indeed, the best service I wish for this book is that it may introduce its readers to that masterpiece of thought and expression, the *Principles of Psychology*. I owe also a personal debt for unfailing kindness and encouragement which can only be acknowledged, never repaid.

PREFACE FOR TEACHERS

This book is designed to serve as a text-book for students who have had no previous training in psychology, who will not in nine cases out of ten take any considerable amount of advanced work in psychology, and who need psychological knowledge and insight to fit them to study, not the special theories of philosophy, but the general facts of human nature. For such students training in methods and technique alone is almost futile: they are not to be expert psychologists, but intelligent men and women. Training in the analysis of the process of thought is equally inadequate: they need more than an introduction to logic and philosophy. A course which reduces psychology to a mass of technical words and definitions is criminal: it hides realities from the student and either encourages him in verbal quibbling or destroys all interest in the study of mental facts. It is the right and the duty of the psychologist as a thinker to specialize, to be an experimentalist, or analyst, or comparative psychologist. But it is the right of the student in a general course on psychology to demand a fair representation of the science as a whole. This book is therefore eclectic in subject matter and in method. Description, definition, analysis, experimentation, comparative and genetic studies—no one of these can wisely be omitted.

This book represents no particular kind of psychology peculiar to the author, nor any radical departures from the general usage of modern text-books on psychology. Some of its features do, however, vary from those of the *elementary* text-books and so deserve comment.

The description of the brain and sense organs follows the recent views instead of those current in the early eighties. By thus discarding the unprofitable geography of 'convolutions,' 'centers' and 'tracts' and utilizing the real facts of the constitution of the nervous system, we not only give the student knowledge of a truly explanatory sort which he can apply to psychological facts, but also supplant an incoherent mass of detail by a simple and clear hypothesis. The length in pages of Part II is due to the photographs and drawings and represents a shortening rather than a lengthening of the student's time and effort.

The descriptive or structural psychology has been sharply separated from the dynamic psychology. For instance, instead of taking up in one chapter both the nature of percepts and the laws of mental action involved in perception and illusion, I have put the latter in Part III along with such topics as instinct, habit and the association of ideas. The older custom is a relic of the 'faculty psychology' and inevitably disposes the student to believe that perception, memory, reasoning and the like are subtle dynamic forces acting on mental processes. By the separation the real value of the terms, sensations, percepts, images, memories, judgments, emotions and the like,—namely, their value as terms describing qualitative differences,—is preserved. Needless to say, the newer arrangement is not only truer to the facts, but also more teachable.

Dynamic psychology is given a place in this book more in accord with the place it holds in present psychological thought than is customary in elementary books. It is surely wise to give adequate space to the facts and laws of instinct, capacity, habit, discrimination, analysis, assimilation, pre-perception, the association of ideas, selective thinking, ideo-motor action and choice. They are the least technical but at the same time the best organized and most instructive topics in psychology.

In one particular the author abandons the accepted doctrine of the psychology books. That images of the resident or remote sensations produced by a movement should be the usual excitant to the movement, he cannot believe and has never taught. In the view presented in the text he has the support of the opinions reached by Kirkpatrick, Woodworth and Bair in the course of actual investigations of voluntary action. The text states frankly that the majority of psychologists believe otherwise.

The exercises and experiments are intended to serve the purpose, not of interesting puzzles or theses to be argued, but rather that served by the problems of the algebra or physics book, by the sentence-writing of a text-book in Latin or French, and by the experiments and demonstrations of a course in chemistry. They are to give the student some very definite thing to do, which he can do, and which can be definitely corrected or approved by the instructor. It is difficult to get such definite material for study and practice in the mental sciences other than logic, but it is a prime necessity for successful teaching, especially in large classes.

The sharp division of the book into descriptive psychology, physiological psychology and dynamic psychology makes some difficulty in the selection of reference readings. Strictly parallel readings are impossible in the case of many chapters. It is on the whole best to follow Professor Titchener's advice and have the class first master one coherent account of the subject and then read one or more other elementary text-books and later still, if there is time, parts of some general treatise. A list of references for individual study of special topics is given at the end of the book.

Teachers College, Columbia University, January, 1905.

PREFACE TO SECOND EDITION

The changes from the first edition consist of alterations of form, especially in the case of the exercises, which the experience of teachers who have used the book recommends. The content remains practically identical with that of the first edition. The reference lists are improved by the utilization of the psychological literature of the past two years. Since an excellent English version of the fifth edition of Wundt's *Physiologische Psychologie* is now progressing toward completion, the references to it have been changed to fit the fifth, instead of the fourth, edition.

Teachers College, Columbia University, December, 1906.

CONTENTS

INTRODUCTION

CHAPTER I

THE SUBJECT MATTER AND PROBLEMS OF PSYCHOLOGY

PART I

DESCRIPTIVE PSYCHOLOGY

CHAPTER II

FEELINGS OF THINGS AND QUALITIES AS PRESENT: SENSATIONS AND PERCEPTS

CHAPTER III

FEELINGS OF THINGS AS ABSENT: IMAGES AND MEMORIES

CHAPTER IV

FEELINGS OF FACTS: FEELINGS OF RELATIONSHIPS, MEANINGS AND JUDGMENTS

CHAPTER V

Feelings of Personal Conditions: Emotions

CHAPTER VI

Mental States Concerned in the Direction of Conduct: Feelings of Willing

CHAPTER VII

General Characteristics of Mental States

CHAPTER VIII

The Functions of Mental States

PART II

The Physiological Basis of Mental Life: Physiological Psychology

CHAPTER IX

The Constitution of the Nervous System

CHAPTER X

The Action of the Nervous System

CHAPTER XI

The Nervous System and Mental States

PART III

Dynamic Psychology

CHAPTER XII

Original Tendencies to Connections

CHAPTER XIII

The Law of Association

CHAPTER XIV

The Law of Dissociation or Analysis

CHAPTER XV

The Connections Between Sense Stimuli and Mental States: Connections of Impression

CHAPTER XVI

The Connections Between One Mental State and Another

CHAPTER XVII

The Connections Between One Mental State and Another (*Continued*)

CHAPTER XVIII

The Connections Between Mental States and Acts: Connections of Expression

CHAPTER XIX

Movements

CHAPTER XX

Selective Processes

CONCLUSION

CHAPTER XXI

The Relations of Psychology

The Elements of Psychology

CHAPTER I

THE SUBJECT MATTER AND PROBLEMS OF PSYCHOLOGY

§ 1. *Mental Facts*

The world is made up of physical and mental facts. On the one hand there are solids, liquids and gases, plants, trees and the bodies of animals, the stars and planets and their movements, the winds and clouds, and so on through the list of physical things and their movements. On the other hand are the thoughts and feelings of men and of other animals; ideas, opinions, memories, hopes, fears, pleasures, pains, smells, tastes, and so on through the list of states of mind. Physics, chemistry, astronomy, botany, zoölogy, geology and the other physical sciences deal with the former group of facts. Psychology, the science of mental facts or of mind, deals with the latter. Human psychology deals with the thoughts and feelings of human beings and seeks to explain the facts of intellect, character and personal life. How do you remember where you were a year ago? Why do we attend to certain sights and sounds and neglect others? What is the difference between an intelligent pupil and an idiot? What decides how large one shall judge an object to be? What happens when a student reasons out a problem in geometry? Such are the questions which the science of psychology tries to answer.

These questions center about four leading topics:

(1) The nature of the different kinds of thoughts and feelings.

(2) The purposes which they serve in life.
(3) The ways in which they are related to the action of the brain or nervous system.
(4) The laws which govern their behavior and that of the bodily states and acts connected with them.

E.g., psychology should give information about:—

(1) Just what attention is.
(2) In what way fear or pain is useful in the conduct of life.
(3) How softening of the brain produces idiocy or how fever produces mental confusion.
(4) Why thinking of one thing makes one think of a certain other thing, or why practice makes perfect.

Its task thus concerns the description of mental states or processes, their function in nature, their relation to the nervous system and the general explanation of the part played by the mind in human life.

Exercises

1. Which of the following words refer to mental facts? Which refer to physical facts? Which refer sometimes to mental and sometimes to physical facts?

Gas, tree, sympathy, money, desire, wish, dog, stone, dreams, headache, inventiveness, inch, pound, taste, intelligence, heavy, sour, oxygen, electricity, fatigue, pleasure, loud, observe, remember, image, teeth.

2. Under which topic, of (1), (2), (3) and (4) above, does each of the following questions belong?

a. Is the fact that a thing gives pleasure a sign that it is good for us?

b. What good does dreaming do?

c. What is the difference between anger and hate?

d. Why are certain people bad spellers in spite of much study?

e. Why is it so much easier to say the alphabet forward than backward?

f. Why does great sorrow make one unconscious of what goes on about him?

g. What are the causes of exceptional musical ability?
h. What are the causes of insanity?
i. What feelings guide us to self-preservation?
j. What feelings guide us to help other people to keep alive?
k. In what respects are imagining and remembering alike?

3. Which of the four aspects of psychology does each of the definitions of psychology given below emphasize?

a. "Psychology is the Science of Mental Life, both of its phenomena and their conditions." (W. James).

b. . . . "We note their resemblances, differences and other relations [the author is speaking of thoughts and feelings] and can thus coördinate them, place under one head those that are alike, and give them a name by which to speak of them." (J. McCosh).

c. "What these phenomena [thoughts and feelings] actually are, as conscious states and how they come to exist and follow each other in the order which they in fact assume, forms the primary subject of the investigations of psychology." (G. T. Ladd).

d. The science of psychology attempts "(1) to analyze concrete (actual) mental experience into its simplest components, (2) to discover how these elements combine, what are the laws which govern their combination, and (3) to bring them into connection with their physiological [bodily] conditions." (E. B. Titchener).

e. "The business of psychology is to furnish a systematic and coherent account of the flow of psychical process in its various forms, phases, and stages, and of the conditions on which it depends." (G. F. Stout).

§ 2. *A General View of Mental States*

The Classification of Mental States.—A list of all the different kinds of thoughts and feelings that human beings have would exceed in length a list of the hundreds of thousands of animals and plants. For convenience psychology divides this total group of mental conditions into a few great classes.

For instance, the feelings of joy, grief, anger, fear,

sympathy and merriment, are alike among themselves in that each is a feeling, not of something in the outside world, but of some personal attitude or condition. All these and similar feelings are grouped together for study, the name used by psychologists in referring to the group being *emotions.* When you close your eyes and call up in imagination your father's face, or your room at home, when you call up the voice of a friend or the melody of a familiar song, you feel in each case some thing or condition, *but as not present.* All such feelings of things, qualities and conditions as not present are grouped together for study under the name *mental images.* To take another instance, the sound of a bell that you hear in a dream, the faces which the fever-patient sees in his delirium, the ghosts which still exist for the mind's eye, may all be classed together since they are all feelings of things as present when really nothing of the sort is actually present. Such feelings are called *hallucinations.*

Some of the chief groups into which thoughts and feelings are classified are:—

1. Sensations.
2. Percepts.
3. Mental Images.
4. Memories.
5. Feelings of Meaning.
    a. concepts or general notions.
    b. individual notions.
    c. abstractions.
6. Feelings of Relationships.
7. Judgments.
8. Emotions.
9. Feelings concerned in the direction of conduct; states of will.

Definitions of These Groups.—The exact nature of

these groups will be made clear in later sections. For the present it will be sufficient to get a rough general idea of them. This can be done easily by making actual observations as follows:—

1. Sit near a hot stove.
   Touch yourself with a pencil.
   Bend your finger.
   Prick yourself with a pin.
   Listen to the tap of a stick on the floor.
   Hold a book at arm's length for one minute.

The feelings of warmth, touch, movement, pain, sound, strain or fatigue and others like them are called *Sensations*. Sensations are feelings of qualities or conditions either of things or of one's own body.

2. Look at a picture.
   Listen to a chord or melody.
   Take hold of a key.

You feel in each case some 'thing' that is present. Such feelings of things present are called *Percepts*.

3. Imagine to yourself the tune of Yankee Doodle.
   Imagine the feeling of velvet.
   Imagine the sight of the moon.
   Imagine that your arm is swinging back and forth.

The feelings you have of the sound, the velvet, the moon and the arm-motion are called *Mental Images*. A mental image is the feeling of a thing or quality or condition when it is really not there and is felt not to be there.

4. Think what you were doing yesterday at one o'clock. Think of what you ate for dinner day before yesterday. Recall the feeling you have when you meet some one whom at first you do not remember but finally remember as having been with you at a certain place. These feelings are called *Memories*.

The term memories is also at times used to include mental images. Thus if any one calls to mind the way his father looks, he may be said either to have a mental image of his father or to remember his father. The words memory and remember and forget are also used for habits or matters of skill that are permanent. Thus we say that we remember how to dance, swim or play the piano. A better name here would be *'the permanence of habits.'*

5. If you have such thoughts as,

   'Eggs are nutritious.'
   'Girls are better than boys.'
   'Electricity is not a fluid.'
   'All teachers should be paid.'
   'Shakspere was a genius.'
   'Virtue is its own reward.'
   'Honesty is the best policy,'

there may be images of sight or sound in connection with the thought but they vary with different people and are not the important thing in the thought. The important thing is the feeling of your *Meaning*. Thus, in the fourth thought, you feel that you mean *all* teachers, though you may have an image of some one teacher, or of the sound of the word 'teacher,' or of something different. These feelings of *Meaning* are very important in all higher sorts of thinking. When the feeling is that we mean every one of a class of things (*e. g.*, 'all teachers', or 'girls') the feeling is called a *general notion or concept.* When we feel that we mean one particular thing (*e. g.*, when we think 'Shakspere' or 'Napoleon' or 'this apple') the feeling is called an *individual notion.* When the feeling is that we mean some element or quality or characteristic apart from the thing or person possessing it, the feeling is called an *abstract idea* or *abstraction.*

6. We feel not only qualities, conditions, objects and meanings, but also the relations between them. *E. g.*, look at two books, one of which is bigger than the other. You feel not only the books, but also their relation of inequality. When you feel 'cats *and* dogs' you have not only two general notions, but also the feeling that the things they mean are to be taken together. 'Cats *without* dogs' would be felt to mean something quite different. Very important among such *Feelings of Relationships* are those of likeness and difference and of cause and effect. Try to observe in yourself the feelings you have when you think of *or, nevertheless, above, below, like, unlike, equal, unequal, the same as,*

7. The entire feelings which you had in thinking the sentences given to show feelings of meaning, would be called *Judgments.* They are feelings that such and such a state of affairs exists, feelings that may be expressed in declarative sentences.

8. The nature of the *Emotions* was briefly described in the second paragraph of § 2. The following list of sample emotions may serve further to define the group:—Admiration, amusement, anger, annoyance, anxiety, awe, envy, fear, gratitude, hatred, joy, love, pity, regret, relief, remorse, restraint, revenge, self-complacency, shame, shyness, sorrow, surprise, suspense, suspicion, sympathy, wonder.

9. Notice your feelings of desire, choice, decision, effort, conflict, impulses and intentions. These feelings and others concerned with action are commonly called *States* of *Will,* or *Volitional States.*

A long list could be made of kinds of feelings which fall more or less outside of these chief groups. *E.g.*, there are feelings of attention, inattention, ennui, interest, belief, uncertainty, inference, etc., etc.

Complex Mental States.—No absolute and sharp classification can be made. It is not necessary or even wise to make a cut-and-dried classification of all thoughts and feelings, since in the ordinary course of mental life mixtures of different kinds of mental states are the common occurrences. *E.g.*, one thinks of a man and at the same time has feelings of attention to the mental image and of aversion toward the man, and perhaps a judgment that he is dishonest. Memory image, attentiveness, emotion and judgment thus combine. Nearly all mental states are pervaded by a feeling of selfhood, by sensations of one's own bodily condition and by a general feeling-tone of well-being or ill-being. It is, however, profitable in studying human nature to analyze complex states of mind into their component parts, to study separately the simpler aspects or parts of the total thought or feeling.

Intermediate Mental States.—It is also true that in the richness of an actual human mind's life there exist very many mental states which do not fall readily into one class rather than another. *E. g.*, is the sound of a bell ringing a sensation or a percept, a feeling of a quality or of a thing? Is the feeling of impatience an emotion or a state of will? Shall the feeling of effort or strain that one has as one holds the mind to a disagreeable task be called a sensation or an emotion? Just as there are some things which may be called either animals or plants, just as there are some streams which are equally well classified as brooks or as rivers,—so there are in mental life intermediate, halfway stages between sensation and perception, perception and image, sensation and state of will, etc. It would be misleading to suppose that a man's mind was by nature divided up into a number of neat bundles, one of sensations, one of percepts, and the like, and that each bundle was quite distinct and separate from all the rest. The division is not absolute, but is like that made when a city is divided into a Chinese quarter, Italian quarter, Jewish quarter, and the like. The divisions grade into each other imperceptibly.

Exercises

1. In studying which of the following studies does one make the most use of (a) the emotions, (b) feelings of meaning, (c) percepts, (d) states of will?—Botany, Music, Grammar, Literature?

2. What kind of a mental fact is referred to by each sentence, except (h), in the following passages?—

(a) "An unaccountable dread seized him. (b) He heard only the rustle of the wind in the trees. (c) Before his mind's eye came a vision of the man whom he had been compelled to forsake. (d) Halting between the choice from two apparently equal evils, he could make up his mind neither to go forward nor to return. (e) 'I shall lose in any case,' he mused."

(f) "In utter amazement, Silas fell on his knees and bent his head low to examine the marvel: (g) it was a sleeping child a round, fair thing, with soft yellow rings all over its head. (h) Could this be his little sister come back to him in a dream—his little sister whom he had carried about in his arms for a year before she died, when he was a small boy without shoes or stockings? (i) But along with that question, and almost thrusting it away, there was a vision of the old home and the old streets leading to Lantern Yard—and within that vision another, of the thoughts which had been present with him in those far-off scenes." (*Silas Marner.*)

3. Which sort of mental fact is usually expressed by a proper noun? By an interjection? By a preposition?

4. What varieties of mental states may verbs express? Give an illustration in each case.

5. Give illustrations of a noun expressing a percept, as when a baby says 'Man, Man'; of a noun expressing a general notion, as when one says, 'Men are mortal'; of a noun expressing an emotion, as when one says, 'Man alive!'

§ 3. *A General View of Human Action*

Since the majority of human actions are directly connected with thoughts or feelings, psychology deals with not only the mental states, but also the acts or conduct of men.

Conduct Equals Movements and Their Connections.—All acts are reducible to movements of the body brought about by the contraction and relaxation of muscles. The common notion of an act, however, includes, besides the mere act itself, the thoughts and feelings leading to it and the circumstances under which it occurs. Thus we commonly regard Caesar's crossing the Rubicon as an act of unique importance, although the act itself was really only a series of alternate muscular contractions identical with the act of going to breakfast. The mere act of saying 'Yes' is the same whether it be a slice of bread or a husband that is accepted. The million things a man does from birth to death are at bottom only some thousands of muscular contractions. A comparatively small number of movements make up the infinite variety of human conduct by being combined in different ways, caused by different feelings and employed in different circumstances. Thus the movements of speech are only varied enough to produce some hundreds of sounds, degrees of loudness and qualities of pitch and timbre, but these few elementary movements combine to produce hundreds of languages, each with thousands of words, capable of making millions of statements and questions, each of which may be an act of many differing meanings according to the intentions and circumstances of its utterance. Human conduct is then made up of (1) *acts proper*, or *movements*, and (2) *the connections between these movements and the various circumstances of life.*

The Classification of Movements.—The common classifications of acts, as right and wrong, conscious and unconscious, normal and abnormal, and the like, are classifications not of acts proper, but of the circumstances under which they occur. The same movement—*e. g.*, winking,—may of course be now right, now wrong, now conscious, now unconscious.

Acts proper or movements may be classified in three ways:—(1) according to their *composition,* (2) according to their *location,* and (3) according to their *function* or *use.* The last is the classification of importance to psychology.

1. Movements are *simple* or *complex.* A complex movement is one that is made up of simpler movements. A simple movement is one that is not.

2. Movements are *hand*-movements, *eye*-movements, *chest*-movements, etc.

3. Movements are *physiological, expressive* and *effective.* Movements of physiological function, such as those involved in swallowing, in the contraction of the heart, in the peristalis of the intestines, or in the expansion of the lungs, have as their chief direct function *to keep the body alive.*

   Movements of expression, such as those involved in laughing, crying, staring and groaning, have as their chief direct function *to reveal inner conditions,—states of mind.*

   Movements of effect, such as those involved in running, striking, grasping and dropping, have as their chief direct function *to bring about results in things or persons.*

Exercises

1. Describe cases in which the same movement results from several different mental states.

2. Describe cases in which the same mental state results in several different movements.

3. Describe cases in which four or five movements result in ten or twelve different actions (in the common meaning of the word) according to the ways in which the movements are connected.

4. Classify the following acts into acts of physiological function, acts of expression and acts of effect: (a) wrinkling the forehead, (b) lifting the arm, (c) curling the fingers in, (d) sneezing, (e) coughing, (f) walking, (g) pushing, (h) raising the eye-brows.

5. Into which of the three classes mentioned in the fourth question would (a) movements of the arms generally fall? (b) Movements caused by facial muscles? (c) Movements of the stomach?

§ 4. *A General View of the Connections of Mental Facts*

The Classification of Mental Connections.—The stuff out of which a human life is made is mental states and movements. What sort of a life it shall be depends upon: first, what mental states and movements compose it, and second, how these are connected. To understand a man's intellect we must know not only what thoughts and feelings he has, but also in what circumstances, that is, in what connections, he has them: to understand his character we must know not only what are his acts, but also in what connection he performs them. All men feel love: the question is *what* they love. All men drink: the difference between the total abstainer and the drunkard lies in the stimulus that provokes the act of drinking. Psychology, to study human life fully, must study not only mental states and bodily acts, but also their connections. And since both thoughts and movements are aroused by events in the physical world[1] which stimulate the organs of sense, psychology must study also the connections between (1) processes in the sense organs and (2) mental states or movements.

The connections to be studied are then:—

(1) Connections between processes in the sense organs and a thought or feeling.

(1a) Connections between processes in the sense organs and a movement.

(2) Connections between one thought or feeling and another.

(3) Connections between a thought or feeling and a movement.

E. g., feeling hot when one goes near the fire is a case of (1): for it is a connection between the outside event, rapid molecular motion, and our sensation of heat. The contractions of the stomach when it contains food illustrate (1a). Thinking of C when one thinks of A B is a case of (2). Going to get food when one becomes hungry is a case of (3).

Connections between Movements and Mental States.—One might expect to study also connections between a movement and a mental state and between one movement and another, but as a matter of fact, movements do not arouse mental states or other movements directly, but only by first connecting with some happening in a sense organ. The (1a) group of connections (between a stimulation of a sense organ and a movement) are more properly a part of physiology than of psychology, since they do not involve any mental fact. I shall therefore not discuss them further.

[1] Thus pressure on the body makes one feel pain; rapid molecular motion makes one feel warm; certain chemical conditions in the body make one feel hungry.

Unlearned and Learned Connections.—Each of these three divisions may be subdivided into:—

A. Unlearned or original or native connections.

B. Learned or acquired connections.

The former are called instincts; the latter, habits. The connection between a blow and a pain is already made in us apart from experience or training (1A), while the connection between the presence of the letters *dog* on a page and the thought of the familiar domestic animal has to be acquired by experience, has to be learned (1B). So also for the connections between a sweet taste and the act of sucking (3A), and the thought 'I have only two minutes to catch the train' and the act of running (3B). The second group of connections are in nearly all, if not in all, cases acquired. That between the thought of the discovery of America and the thought of Columbus is a sample.

Classes (1), (2), and (3) may be called connections of *Impression, Association* and *Expression* respectively. There are then:—

(1A) Native or unlearned connections of impression.
(1B) Acquired or learned connections of impression.
(?) (2A) Native or unlearned connections of association.
(2B) Acquired or learned connections of association.
(3A) Native or unlearned connections of expression.
(3B) Acquired or learned connections of expression.

Each of the six classes so far made could be subdivided again to almost any extent according to the kind of outside events, mental states and bodily movements involved. Thus (2B), acquired habits of association, could be divided into associations between sensations and concepts, images and emotions, images and images, emotions and impulses, judgments and judgments, etc.

In the case of class (3) it is useful to subdivide also according to the extent to which the connection of the bodily act with the feeling is modified and controllable. Some connections (*e.g.*, the contraction of the pupil of the eye in response to the brightness of the light) cannot be altered. Others, forming the great majority, can (*e. g.*, grasping certain objects in response to seeing them).

Further Classification.—The following names used in psychology books for certain kinds of connections need explanation either because they are technical terms or are common words used with a special meaning:—Reflexes, Instincts, Habits, Powers, Capacities, Associations of Ideas, Inferences, Reasonings.

Reflexes include those connections of events in the body,—sometimes felt in sensation, sometimes not,—with movements, in which the act follows the impression automatically, without either intention or control on our part (*e. g.*, turning in the toes when the sole of the foot is tickled, the contraction of the pupil of the eye in response to light, or sneezing when the membrane of the nose is irritated).

Instincts, as now commonly defined, include reflexes and all other connections or tendencies to connections amongst thoughts, feelings and acts which are unlearned, —are in us apart from training or experience. Anything that we do without having to learn to do it, in brief, is an instinct. Thus, crying when pain is felt, starting at a sudden noise, feeling fear at large, strange, moving objects seen in the dark, feeling anger when food is snatched away from one and laughing when tickled, are instincts of babyhood; to feel jealousy when rivalled by one of the same sex and to act conspicuously when attracted by one of the opposite sex, are instincts of youth. The common usage of the words instinct and instinctive differs from the psychologist's usage. People commonly say that they do or feel certain things instinctively when they act or feel without deliberation or forethought or clear consciousness of what or why; *e. g.,* "He instinctively lifted the glass to his lips." "By instinct I realized that the only way of escape was directly through the fire." Neither of these cases would be called instinctive by the psychologist. For to him an instinct means an act that is the result of mere inner growth, not of training or experience.

Habits.—Tendencies to respond which are created in whole or in part by experience, practice or training are called *Habits.* The instinctive tendencies become habits as soon as experience alters them. Practically all of human behavior is a series of illustrations of habits. In common talk the word is used only of tendencies to respond which have become *very* frequent and *very* habitual, such as eating three meals a day, taking off our clothes when we go to bed, bowing to acquaintances, thinking four when we see 2+2, and the like. But the essential nature of the behavior is the same whether the habit is partially formed and rarely used or fully formed and always used. Indeed, for psychology every tendency for anything to go with anything else is either a case of a pure instinct or of habit.

Powers.—Habits not in action and possibilities of forming habits are called *Powers.* For instance, that man has the power to avoid theft who would be habitually honest, though tempted, or who will habitually, when tempted, not thieve.

Capacities.—The inborn qualities which are the partial basis for the development of mental powers might be called instincts of possibility rather than of fact, they being qualities which will result in the presence of the powers or habits corresponding to them when the proper circumstances arise. The common word for these instincts of possibility is *Capacities.* Thus the capacity for composing music means the qualities which, though themselves unknown, will, when the proper opportunity comes, blossom out into the power to compose music and the habit of doing so.

Associations of Ideas.—Those habits of thought by which any one state of mind tends to call up another state of mind are called *Associations of Ideas.* Thus we should say that the thought of AB calling up the thought of C, or the thought of 90 degrees calling up the thought of heat or of a right angle, were cases of the association of ideas, or, more clearly, of habits in the realm of ideas.

Inferences.—When one thought or judgment calls up another leading on to some related conclusion the process is called an *Inference.* Thus, whereas we would call the sequence, 'John is sick. I like John,' a mere association of ideas, we should regard as an inference the sequence, 'John has the measles. Fred has been playing with him. Fred will probably have the measles.' A series of such directed thoughts or inferences is called *Reasoning* or *Rational Thinking.*

In general the term *Situation* is used for any total set of circumstances in the outside world and in one's body by which the mind is influenced; *Stimulus* is used for any particular part of a situation; *Reaction* and *Response* are used for the act, and sometimes for the mental state, that occurs as a result of the stimulus.

Exercises

1. Classify the following cases of connection as (1A), (1B), (2A), (2B), (3A) or (3B), or at least as (1), (2) or (3).

a. Shutting the eyes when a bright light is flashed into them.
b. Bowing to an acquaintance seen.
c. Hearing ten times eight and thinking eighty.
d. Seeing a pin and picking it up.
e. Feeling pain at a severe blow.
f. Thinking of an engagement at a distance and taking one's hat and coat and starting.
g. Thinking of 'I cannot tell a lie' and then of George Washington.
h. Feeling disbelief at seeing, "England has voted to do away with the King and the House of Lords."
i. Seeing red when light waves of 460 billion vibrations per second strike the retina of the eye, and violet when the waves have a vibration rate of 790 billions per second.
j. Thinking of 8 after thinking 1, 2, 3, 4, 5, 6, 7.

2. Which of the cases above are reflexes? Which are associations of ideas?

3. Why might ideo-motor connections or ideo-motor actions be a suitable name for d and f?

4. Name two connections between a mental state and a bodily act which are acquired. Two that are unlearned or native.

5. What are some common connections between thoughts that are acquired in the study of arithmetic? In the study of Latin? Of what sort are the connections formed in learning to play the piano?

6. Give cases illustrating the difference between mere association of ideas and inference.

7. Name two or three beneficial instincts. Two or three undesirable ones.

References

A. James, *Briefer Course,* I., XXIII.
Stout, *Manual,* 1-14, 56-70.
Titchener, *Outline,* §§ 1-4, 61.

B. Ebbinghaus, *Grundzüge,* §§ 1, 2, 3, 12.
James, *Principles,* I., XXIII.
Wundt, *Physiologische Psychologie,* Einleitung (or, *Principles of Physiological Psychology,* Introduction).

PART I

DESCRIPTIVE PSYCHOLOGY

CHAPTER II

Feelings of Qualities and Things as Present: Sensations and Percepts

The topic of this and of the next five chapters will be the nature of the different groups of mental states. These six chapters may be grouped together under the general title, **Descriptive Psychology.**

§ 5. *The Nature of Sensations*

Definitions.—The word *Sensations* is used by writers of psychology with several different meanings. Sometimes they include under this term only feelings of brightness, color, size, pitch, loudness, timbre or tone-quality, taste, smell, touch, pressure, resistance, movement, heat, cold, pain, position, rotation, hunger, thirst and other feelings of definite qualities of things and well known conditions of the body. But often they include also the feelings of fatigue of different sorts, of effort or strain, of suspense or expectancy, of shock, shuddering, trembling, well-being, malaise, dizziness and other feelings of vague and little understood bodily conditions.

Ordinarily they include only the simple, bare, uncombined feelings under the term sensation and treat the actual complex feelings (*e.g.,* of the taste of a mouthful of acid, the smell of the woods or the touch of a pin, as mixtures or combinations of simpler elementary feelings. But they also use the word more vaguely for all direct feelings of the qualities of things or of conditions of the body which are not the definite feelings of things classed as percepts or the rich combinations of feelings classed as emotions. This being the usage, the complex sound of a city street, the taste of coffee or the shock of a cold plunge would be called a sensation. Sensations are sometimes defined as the primitive, bare elements of mental life, the first things in consciousness. From this point of view only the original appearance of any feeling may be called sensation; after that the mental state equals sensation plus association or experience.

The fact of importance that appears from these various definitions, is that they and all others are arbitrary, that in fact we cannot draw clear lines of distinction between sensations of qualities of things and sensations of bodily conditions,—between sensations from special, well-known stimuli like sounds and from vague, ill-known stimuli like the condition of the blood or the gnawings of dyspepsia,—between atomic, indivisible bits or brightness or pain or bitter and complex masses of color, toothache or tones,—between the first sensation of any sort and the subsequent ones modified by it. Nor can we draw a clear line around sensations (taken in the broad sense shown by the group of samples above) so as to infallibly separate sensations from percepts or from emotions or from certain feelings of relationships. It is indeed as important to know that these mental states shade off the one into the other as to know the general features of difference which lead us to separate them into groups.

Realizing then that definitions must be rough, one

may say that *sensations are direct feelings of qualities of things or of conditions of the body. Pure sensations are such feelings when uninfluenced by previous experiences. Elementary sensations are such feelings so simple or minute as to be unanalyzable into simpler ones.*

Pure Sensations.—Except in the first experiences of early infancy, pure sensations are not found. The ways in which the outside world and our own bodily states are felt are the result of original tendencies combined with practice. Thus artists who wish to get back to the bare, immediate sizes and colors of things, apart from the influence of our habitual interpretations of them, have to undergo special training to free themselves from the, for their purposes, disadvantageous tendencies of experience. Although in actual mental life pure sensations are not found, it is possible in thought to regard any sensation as a pure sensation plus the modifications in it due to experience, and to argue about the pure sensation's factor or share or aspect by itself.

Elementary Sensations. — Elementary sensations are not real fragments of our mental states, but abstractions invented to aid our understanding of mental life. They exist in the sense that lines without breadth or thickness exist. Just as an actual boundary wall is not a sum of such lines, so the sensations we have are not sums or collections of tiny atomic sensations. An intense salt taste is not the sum of a thousand slightly salt tastes, any more than the thought of a chair is the thought of *c* plus the thought of *h* plus the thought of *a* and so on. Our feelings of the outside world can in thought be analyzed into elements of colors, sounds, pressures and the like, but in actual experience they are felt as complex total feelings. Nor does the mind in its sense life grow from a starting-point of elementary sensations by the addition of more and more of them and by building them into complex wholes. On the contrary, the first sensations are extremely vague, rich, complicated feelings of comfort, discomfort, bodily disturbances and such appearances of external things as are well characterized by Professor James' phrase 'a big, blooming, buzzing confusion.' The progress of the mind is by the differentiation of vague feelings into more and more definite and detailed feelings. The clean-cut reds and blues, A flats and C sharps, sweets and sours, hards and softs which we call elementary sensations are the result of slow growth. The world of sense comes not as a building constructed of small pieces of bricks and mortar and glass, but as a landscape gradually clearing up from the obscurity of a fog. The child comes to feel hot, cold, red and green as we come to distinguish the constituents of a salad-dressing, the sounds of the different instruments in an orchestra, or the characteristic odors of a slum.

It is nevertheless desirable to try to analyze any actual sensation into, or replace it in thought by such fictitious elements. Fictitious in the sense of being elements of mental states which when put together give the sensation, they are real in the sense of corresponding to elementary processes in the brain which, when happening together, *do* produce in mental life the sensation. The sensation produced in the mind when one plunges the hand into cold water is not the equivalent of a thousand feelings of little cold spots plus a thousand feelings of little slipperinesses and elasticities, but the brain process which produces the feeling of a cold and wet hand is the equivalent of thousands of component processes.

The Attributes of Sensations.—Every sensation, and indeed every mental state of any sort, is in time, lasts so long, possesses *Duration* as an attribute.

Every sensation possesses *Intensity,* by which we mean that there is a certain amount of it which can be conceived to have possibly been more or less.

That every sensation is felt as possessing *Bigness* or *Extensity* is held to be true by some psychologists. Others would limit the attribute of spatial quality more narrowly; *e.g.,* to sensations from the eyes and skin and joints. Others even deny it to all sensations, arguing that by itself a sensation is felt as nowhere and of no size, that only in the connection of many sensations with one another does the feeling of 'thereness' and 'voluminousness' appear. Those announcing this third view presumably refer only to elementary sensations.

Every sensation possesses *Quality,* which can be defined provisionally by examples: color, pitch and sweetness are qualities of sensations.

If anyone examines his own sensations, he will find that they may differ from one another in these four ways: One may last a longer or shorter time than another; may be more or less vigorous or intense; may be bigger or smaller; *i.e.,* may fill more or less space; may be different in mental stuff, in its very nature. In all but the last case sensations may be ranged in a series according to the *amount* of some attribute they possess; they may be ranked by the *quantity* of time, or energy, or extent belonging to them. The fourth case of differences cannot be expressed as differences of quantity, but only as of the *kind* or *quality* of the feelings. When the differences between sensations fail to resolve themselves into a series of amounts of any one thing they are therefore called differences of *Quality.* Thus with red and green, the touch of velvet and that of soft soap, the feeling of nausea and that of a toothache. The quality of a sensation is thus *the attribute of it which distinguishes it from any other sensation.*

§ 6. *The Classification of Sensations*

By Their Quality.—Sensations may be classified according to their degrees of difference in quality. All colors are more like each other in quality than they are like tastes. All reds are more like each other than they are like blues, but are more like blues than they are like tastes. Touches are more like pressures than they are like smells. We thus classify sensations according to the sense to which they belong.

Within each sense we have further classification; for instance, of sensations of vision into the different colors or of sensations of hearing into noises and tones. Although in the spectrum red shades off into orange, orange into yellow and yellow into green and so on, we feel the change to be more abrupt at certain places than at others and so group color-sensations into reds, oranges, yellows, greens and the like. So also sounds are grouped into noises and tones, though a tone that lasts but a very short time is indistinguishable from a noise and certain combinations of noises, such as the sound of certain machines heard at a distance, take on the likeness of tones.

By the Sense Organs Causing Them.—Sensations are also classified according to the sense organ the activity of which arouses them. Every educated person knows that his feelings of color are due to the influence of light rays upon the visual sense organ, the eye; that his sensations of sound are due to the influence of air vibrations upon the auditory sense organ, the ear. It is equally true that tastes, smells, heat, cold, pressures and other varieties of sensation correspond each to the activity of one kind of sense organ or combination of sense organs. Some of these sense organs,—*e.g.*, the eyes, ears, and nose,— are influenced by stimuli exterior to the body, such as ether vibrations and air vibrations. Some are influenced by stimuli within the body, such as the rubbing of the surfaces of the joints, changes in the blood supply, inflammation of the tissues and the like.

The large groups resulting from a classification on the basis of the sense organs concerned are:—

A. Sensations from the periphery of the body: *External Sensations.*

Sensations from the eyes.
" " " ears.
" " " nose.
" " " mouth.
" " " skin.

B. Sensations from the internal organs of the body: *Internal Sensations.*

Sensations from the semicircular canals in the internal ear.

Sensations from the muscles.
" " " tendons.
" " " surfaces of the joints.
" " " alimentary canal.
" " " circulatory system.
" " " lungs.
" " " brain and nerves themselves.
" " " sex-organs.

Within each of these groups a finer grouping can often be made out. The skin or cutaneous sensations, *e.g.*, are apparently due to different sorts of nerve endings in the skin and may accordingly be divided into feelings of pressure, heat, cold, pain, and perhaps of traction (due to pulling the skin or hairs outward) touch, tickling and others. The mouth is perhaps furnished with four different sorts of nerve-endings, each the source of a special variety of taste (sweet, sour, salt and bitter).

Finally each variety of sense organ may be capable of arousing many different sensations, according to the different ways in which it may behave,—the differences in action of which it is capable. Thus in the retina of the eye the so-called 'rods' and 'cones,' which are the nerve-endings concerned in vision, are apparently each capable of arousing hundreds of different shades of color and degrees of brightness.

In a classification resulting from perfect knowledge, the main classes will correspond to the kind of sense organ involved, the sub-classes to the kinds of activity of each kind of sense organ.

The Two Types of Classification Compared.—With respect to the more obvious and more important groups of sensations the classification on the basis of felt resemblances parallels that on the basis of the sense organ concerned. The differences between the two classifications are due first to the fact that common-sense judgments of qualities often put compound sensations into a single group although they involve very different sense organs. Thus when what common sense calls tastes are found to be due largely to stimulation, not of the gustatory nerve-endings in the mouth, but of the olfactory nerve-endings in the nose,[1] psychology changes popular usage and reserves the word tastes for the bare sweets, sours, salts, bitters (and possibly alkaline and metallic tastes) and classifies the rich savors of foods as smell sensations.

[1] Hence the loss of 'taste' when one has a cold in the head. One can gain experimental evidence of the share of the nose in taste by testing some friend, who with eyes shut and nose carefully plugged, tries to distinguish raw potato from apple, maple syrup from molasses, soup from salt water.

Even expert analysis sees no difference between the sensations from the rods in the retina and those from the cones and has always made a single class,—visual sensations. Yet it is perhaps true that the rods act only when the light is dim, and give no sensations at all for green. On the basis of the sense organ involved a classification into sensations in a dim light and sensations in a bright light would be, perhaps, more scientific and fundamental than one into colors and brightness.

Classifications by felt quality and by known sense organ differ in the second place because clear and important differences can often be felt where no corresponding difference in the nerve-endings involved has been discovered. For example, sweets and sours and bitters deserve separate classes from their felt unlikeness, but no proof of different nerve-endings for each class has yet been offered.

Two general cautions are necessary in connection with the classification of sensations. First, in trying to pick out the different kinds of sensations one should not forget that the actual stream of mental life rarely offers a single kind of sensation at a time. Our feelings of the outside world are feelings of complex things involving many different sensations, or of numerous qualities at the same time. The feeling of a lifted weight, for example, is a complex due to the action of sense organs in the skin, on the surfaces of the joints and in the muscles themselves. Second, the fact that only the more definite and frequent sensations, such as sights, sounds and tastes, are easily classified should not blind one to the existence and importance of the vaguer sensations, such as fatigues, aches, hunger and the like. The condition of the body as a whole, the state of its muscular tension, circulation, digestion, and other obscurer activities, influences the little known internal sense organs, and so causes those mental states which verge from sensations toward emotions. These must not be neglected.

§ 7. *Sensation and Stimulus*

Sensations correspond to and are due to physical causes and happenings without and within the body, which cause activity in the sense-organs. Such a physical cause of activity in a sense-organ is called the *Stimulus* to the sensation.

The *Threshold* of sensibility for any variety of sensation is the least possible stimulus that will cause it, *i.e.*, the softest sound, the weakest light, the slightest touch.

The *Range* of sensibility in any sense is the range of physical stimuli below and above which the stimulus causes no sensation. For instance, the range of pitch is from about 16 vibrations of the air per second to about 30,000 vibrations per second;[1] the range of color vision is from about 450 billion[2] to about 790 billion vibrations of the ether per second;[3] *i.e.*, from the extreme of red to the extreme of violet.

It would be possible, though not in the present condition of knowledge especially useful, to classify sensations by the physical facts which cause them, by the nature of their stimuli. We should then have as the two chief groups:

A. Feelings caused by the qualities of outside objects.

B. Feelings caused by qualities of the body itself.

[1] These figures vary among different individuals, and different values have been assigned to them by different investigators. The low limit is almost certainly between 8 and 30.

[2] A billion means here, following the European usage, a million millions.

[3] Under favorable circumstances a red of only 412 billion vibrations can be distinguished and a color beyond the violet end of the spectrum of 912 billion vibrations. The range varies with individuals as in the case of sound.

Under A we should have:

A I. Feelings caused by light, *i.e.*, by ether vibrations.

A II. Feelings caused by molecular motions.

- A II 1. By tones, *i.e.*, periodic wave motions.
- A II 2. By noises, *i.e.*, non-periodic motions.
- A II 3. By temperature, *i.e.*, inner molecular motions.

A III. Feelings caused by gross mechanical forces.

- A III 1. By weight.
- A III 2. By elasticity.
- Etc.

A VI. Feelings caused by chemical forces.

- A IV 1. In gaseous form (causing sensations of smell).
- A IV 2. In liquid form (causing sensations of of taste).

Under B (feelings caused by qualities of the body itself) the movements of the ether and of sound waves would play a small if not a zero role while electrical forces might perhaps be found to influence feelings as they do not when acting through outside objects. To such classifications on the basis of the nature of the physical stimulus are due the terms: the *chemical senses,* for taste and smell; the *mechanical senses,* for touch, pressure, etc.; the *distant senses,* for vision and hearing.

The richness of the contribution of sensations to mental life hardly requires comment. The number of qualities of things felt in vision or hearing or touch alone or the multitude of bodily conditions of which the organic senses, including pain, warn us, is certainly astounding. The loss of a single sense deprives a human life of a whole kingdom of facts. It is more necessary to call attention to the fact that although the number of the different sensations that a human being feels seems almost infinite, they represent the influence on us of only a part of the world's forces. Sensations are aroused only by a selected few of the events about us and in our bodies. Sounds are due to air waves, but waves above thirty or forty thousand vibrations per second cause no sensations of sound in man, though they apparently do in some insects. The x-rays and the emanations from radio-active bodies cause no sensations directly. All about us there may be forces in nature to which our senses are not susceptible. What we feel are the comparatively few series of stimuli to which our senses are, so to speak, tuned. The growth of tissues, the action of certain glands, and the destruction of dangerous substances by the white blood corpuscles are samples of important events within the body which leave us unfeeling. To only a few of the multitudinous events of our bodily lives are we sensitive. Our sensations warn us of only a fraction of the happenings of the universe within and without.

Exercises

1. Of the feelings referred to in the list of words, phrases or sentences given below which are most like emotions?
2. Which are most like feelings of relationships?
3. Which would be called sensations without any hesitation?
4. Which might possibly be called elementary sensations?
5. Which might possibly be called pure sensations?
6. Which are internal sensations?
7. Which are compounds caused by at least two different senses?

a. The child's feeling when it first burns itself.
b. Hunger.
c. The sound of a tuning fork.
d. The general feeling of being well or ill.
e. The faintest possible taste of bitter.
f. Feelings of weight.

g. Nausea.
h. Feelings of distance.
i. The taste of coffee.
j. An unrecognized smell.
k. The ringing in the ears that results from a large dose of quinine.
l. Sleepiness.
m. Hearing a note sung *crescendo.*
n. Lassitude.
o. Restlessness.
p. The sight of a light by a four-weeks-old baby.

8. Show how the author of the following passage classifies sensations partly on the basis of felt likeness and partly on the basis of the sense organs concerned:

"Different Classes of Sensation.—Passing now to the enumeration and comparison of the different classes of sensation we may begin with the following provisional list: Sensations of sight, of hearing, of contact and pressure; those due to the varying states of muscles, joints, and tendons as dependent on the position and movement of the limbs; sensations of smell, of taste, of temperature, and finally organic sensations. The last head requires some explanation. Under the term 'organic sensation' are included sensations due to the state of the internal organs of the body, such as headache, thirst, muscular cramp, or fatigue, nausea, etc." (G. F. Stout, *Groundwork of Psychology,* p. 42.)

9. Which groups in this classification most need further subdivision.

10. What criticism may be made of a description of a group of feelings as "those due to the varying states of the muscles, joints and tendons as dependent on the position and movement of the limbs"?

11. Criticise the following classification:

"Sensation. There are two classes of sensations,—*General* and *Special.*

General Sensations include all those which do not belong to the "five senses,"—those which constitute our bodily comfort or discomfort; they may be classed as follows:

Muscular Sensations of injury, fatigue, and repose.

Nervous Sensations arising from the state of the nervous system, as when we feel the exhilaration of perfect health or are weakened by care or suffering.

Vital Sensations, depending on the condition of the vital organs, as those of hunger and thirst and their opposites, the pain of indigestion, the feeling of suffocation when breathing impure air.

Special Sensations are of five kinds, namely, those of *Touch* (including those of the *"Muscular Sense"*), *of Sight, of Hearing,* of *Taste,* and of *Smell."*

12. No one has found a classification of smells that is either simple or comprehensive or scientific. It is interesting to try to classify the odors of the objects named below and compare the groups one makes with those made by others:

alcohol	coffee	orange peel
apples	ether	pine woods
bananas	fir balsam	roast beef
benzine	fish (cooked)	roses
cabbage (cooked)	fish (raw)	rubber
camphor	hay	sour milk
canteloupes	kerosene	strawberries
cheese	lemons	sulphur (burning)
chloroform	maple sugar	sulphuretted hydrogen
cinnamon	onions	violets

13. Give the names of two things which seem to you to have somewhat the same kind of a smell that the thing named has, in the case of each of the following:

chloroform	coffee	tobacco
camphor	rancid butter	decaying meat
cinnamon	roses	new mown hay
alcohol	apples	cheese
benzine	onions	bananas

14. Make a list of senses which it is conceivable that human beings might have, though they do not.

15. Which one of the senses provides the greatest variety of different qualities?

16. Which sensations are aroused by distant objects?

17. Which sensations are least delusive, most reliable?

Experiment 1. Pressure Spots.—On the back of the hand, say between the base of the thumb and the base of the forefinger, mark off an area about an inch long and a half inch wide. Have ready: (1) a pyramid of cork about a quarter inch square at the base, about one quarter inch high and cut to a point, with a long needle or a tooth pick stuck into its base for a handle; (2) two small metal rods, such as knitting needles, or pieces of wire with rounded ends, or better two hollow metal cylinders drawn to a closed point at one end.

Go over the surface of the skin with the point of the cork, touching each square millimeter lightly. Note the location of any spots where the touch of the cork arouses a much more pronounced feeling of pressure (of what is commonly called touch) than it does in general. Does the touch of the cork in some spots arouse a feeling of coolness? If so, locate these.

Experiment 2. Cold Spots.—Go over the surface of the skin with one of the rods cooled to say 50° Fahrenheit (if the hollow rods are used, they need only to be filled with cold water) and note the location of any spots where the touch arouses a much more pronounced feeling of coolness than it does in general. Touch these spots with the cork. What sensation results? Touch them with the second rod warmed slightly above the temperature of the room. What sensation results?

As an aid to remembering the location of the pressure spots and cold spots, it will be useful to draw on paper an enlarged outline of the area marked off on the hand, or to mark the hand itself with a tiny spot of ink or paint.

Experiment 3. The Threshold for Pressure.—Make 5 cylinders of wood about 4 millimeters in diameter and 1, 2, 4, 8, and 16 millimeters in height. Have each one smooth at top and bottom. Fasten to the center of the top of each by a bit of glue, a fine, flexible thread of silk. Tie the thread to one end of a small stick (tooth picks will serve), letting the length from the cylinder to the stick be about two inches. Holding the stick at the end removed from the thread, lower the cylinder gradually till it rests on some smooth surface, as a table-top. Each cylinder should, when thus lowered, have the plane of its bottom surface parallel with the table-top.

Let a friend be seated with eyes closed, fore-arm resting on a table, and the palm of the hand upward. Say to him: "I shall give as a signal the word *ready.* Then at the end of two seconds I shall either put a very light weight on your hand or I shall do nothing. If you feel a weight, say 'Yes,' if you do not feel any, say nothing." Then say, 'Ready,' and lower a cylinder gently till it rests on the center of the palm. Note the answer given, and remove the cylinder slowly. Record the answer. Repeat with another and so on through the following series: the 16mm. cyl-

3

inder, the 8, 0 (that is, none at all), 16, 0, 2, 4, 2, 16, 0, 1, 8, 8, 2, 1, 4, 16, 1, 8, 1, 8, 1, 16, 2, 0, 1, 2, 0, 0, 2, 0, 16, 1, 1, 8, 0, 16, 16, 8, 2, 0, 0, 4, 4, 16, 0, 8, 8, 0, 16, 0, 4, 0, 2, 16, 0, 1, 1, 16, 1, 4, 2, 2, 8, 4, 0, 16, 4, 4, 4, 16, 16, 0, 0, 16.

Record the answers by drawing a line under the figure denoting the cylinder used if the subject answers yes, and a line through it if he says nothing. This method of scoring serves also to keep track of which cylinder is the next to be used.

Which weights are below the threshold? (Unless a cylinder was felt in eight cases out of ten it was probably not really sensed at all, for mere guessing would of course give fifty per cent. of correct answers.)

Try the same experiment placing the weights on the back of the wrist or fore-arm. Which weights are below the threshold here?

Experiment 4. The Mixture of Taste and Smell.—Arrange for a friend to give you a half hour of his time. Prepare 4 pieces (cubes about one quarter of an inch long) of each of the following: raw apple, raw onion, raw celery, cooked chicken, cooked beef, cooked lamb; and have ready a half spoonful each of honey, maple syrup, molasses, cinnamon, clove and nutmeg, a medicine dropper (a plain glass rod will do) and a salt spoon or a visiting card cut lengthwise into six or seven strips.

Let the subject of the experiment be seated, with eyes closed and nose carefully plugged with cotton. Say to him, "I shall put something in your mouth; taste it and tell me what it is before you swallow it." Require the subject to answer at once before the odor can penetrate to the nose through the passage at the back of the mouth cavity. Then place a piece or drop or pinch of the food, say a pinch of cinnamon, on his tongue and record his answer. Give the different substances in a mixed-up order, using each two times, and recording the substance and the answer in each case.

After these 24 trials have been made, remove the filling from the subject's nose and repeat the 24 trials.

Compare the number of errors in the two cases. Why would it be desirable to repeat the experiment on another person, testing him first with nose open and later with nose plugged?

References

A. James, *Briefer Course,* II. (9-16), III., IV., V., VI.
   Stout, *Manual,* 117-124, 141-198.
   Titchener, *Outline,* §§ 7-26.
   Angell, *Psychology,* V.

B. Ebbinghaus, *Grundzüge,* §§ 13-36.
   James, *Principles,* XVII. (1-9).
   Wundt, *Physiologische Psychologie,* VII., VIII., X.

§ 8. *Percepts*

The Nature and Attributes of Percepts.—Our consciousness of the world is commonly not of confused blurs and masses of colors, sounds, tastes, and the like, but of unified wholes which we call 'things.' We can in thought analyze our feelings of the outside world into elements of colors, sounds, pressures, etc., but in reality they appear as complex total feelings. The feeling of a 'thing' as actually present is called a *Percept* if the thing is actually present; an *Illusion* if it is not present but something else is which gives us the feeling; an *Hallucination* if nothing is actually present to cause the feeling. Thus my feelings of the page I see, the pen I hold, the chords being played on the piano or the puffing of an engine are percepts. My feelings, as I lie dozing, of a page seen, when really only a dirty blotter is seen, and of the puffing of an engine, when really only my own breathing is heard, are illusions. My feeling of music heard in a dream, when really no sound at all is audible, is an hallucination.

Feelings of things are most commonly based on sight and touch, less commonly on hearing, still less commonly on taste, smell or pain, and almost never on the feelings of nausea, dizziness, muscle-strain and other inner bodily conditions. We rarely say or think, 'I have a sourness,' or 'There are four dizzinesses in this room.'

Percept and Stimulus.—The same outside thing may arouse different percepts, different feelings of it, in different people according to the amount and nature of their previous experiences of it. To the man without musical training the song sung by a chorus is a vague total of sounds, but to the trained musician it is a balanced harmony in which all the different parts are clearly felt. To the five year old a page of print is an indefinite smear of black specks on a white ground; to his teacher it is a definite series of letters and words; to the printer it is not only that, but also 10 point type. To the baby all our 'things' are as yet a misty, chaotic muddle of feeling.

We learn our feelings of the commonest things as truly as we learn the multiplication table or the Latin language. The differences are that we learn the former mainly in the earliest years of life, that the constant presence of things and the need of getting on with them makes the acquaintance with them almost universal and brings to pass far greater similarities amongst men in their percepts than in the more elaborated connections between ideas. These similarities should not, however, blind us to the differences which do, as has been pointed out, exist, or to the fact that even by the age of entrance to school the feelings of things which adults have long taken for granted may be absent or only partially developed.

One of the results of experience is that less and less of the outside thing is required to arouse the feeling of it. Our eyes really see and our ears hear only a part of what we feel as visual and auditory percepts. In all probability a number of readers of this book did not actually see the *of* in the first line of this paragraph or the *the* in the second line or the last *e* of outside. If the reader will read very rapidly the passage printed on page 38 and then re-read it very slowly, looking at each word, he will probably discover that in the first reading his senses must have taken in only partial glimpses of the words and that his mind supplied their customary accompaniments out of whole cloth. In listening to a foreign language one is surprised at the small number of articulate sounds that he hears: the rest seem a mere jangle. Of conversation in our own language our ears really hear only a few sounds clearly, but these serve as a sufficient basis for a total series of clear percepts. Repeat to a group of people the lines below and you may be surprised to find the changes unnoticed.

Mary had a little lamb,
Its fleece was white is snow;
And every pair that Mary went,
The lamb was sure to go.

Percepts and Sensations Compared.—Between sensations and percepts, between feelings of the qualities of things and feelings of the things themselves, no sharp line can be drawn. *E.g.*, is my feeling of the sound of the watch ticking to be called a sensation of the sound, a quality of the watch, or a percept of a thing, a ticking sound? If by sensations are meant what were called pure sensations, the clear distinction can be drawn that every percept involves experience, that 'every perception is an acquired perception.' But since pure sensations exist only in the dawn of mental life, this distinction is as useless as it is clear. Again between elementary sensations and percepts the clear distinction can be drawn that every percept is caused by a number of sensory stimulations, requires the co-operation of many brain processes, is divisible in analysis into parts. But since elementary

We, the people of the United States, in order to form a more perfect union, establish justice, insure domestic tranquillity, provide for the common defence, promote the general welfare, and secure the blessings of liberty to ourselves aud our posterity, do ordain and establish this Constitntion for the United Stales of America.

All legislative powers herein granted shall be vested in a Congress of the United States, which shall consist of a Senate and House of Represcntatives.

The House of Representatives shall be composed of members chosen every second year by the people of the several States, and the electors in each State shall have the qualifications requisite for electors of tho most numerous branch of the State legislature.

No person shall be a Representative who shall not have attained the age of twenty-five years, ard been seven years a citizen of the United States, and who shall not, when elected, be an inhahitant of that State in which he shall be chosen.

Representatives and direct taxes shalt be apportioned among the several States which may be included within this Union, according to their respective numbers, which shall be determimed by adding to the whole number of free persons, including those bound to service for a term of years, and excluding Indians not taxed, threc fifths of all other persons. The actual enumeration shall be made within three years after the first meeting of the Congress of the United States, and within every subsequent term of ten years, in such manner as they shall by law direct.

sensations do not have real existence, it may be objected that there is no great advantage in distinguishing anything from them.

The facts are that *sensations* and *percepts* are words that divide between them the work of naming our feelings of the outside world as present; that in their general use the former refers to our feelings when they emphasize simple qualities such as of color, pitch, heat, cold, and the like, while the latter refers to our feelings when they emphasize things or groups of qualities that go together.

The Classification of Percepts.—There is literally no end to the variety of the feelings of things possible to a human mind. In an hour's walk in a city one may have five thousand different percepts, each of a human face. In an evening at the opera one may add thousands of percepts of tones. A classification in any detail of the perceptual life of a mind would thus be a long labor. There may be as many and as different percepts in the mind as there are things in the world, indeed more. For the same thing may arouse different feelings according as it is seen near or at a distance, in the light or in the dark, from one side or from the other, and so on through many possible changes.

For purposes of study a classification according to which sense furnishes the main features of the percept is useful. Thus we have visual percepts, auditory percepts, etc. The word main must be emphasized in our thought, for in many percepts different senses combine.

Another classification useful for purposes of study would be into *extensive, temporal* and merely *qualitative.* For many of our feelings are of things as in space, as so big, of such a shape, at such a distance, and the spatial or form-size character of things is highly important in the sciences and arts. So also the precepts of language and music in which elements successive in time become joined into unitary feelings of words or melodies well deserve separate study. The group left over—the feeling of things through taste, smell, pressure and the rest —is, however, a very mixed and unwieldy group.

In discussions of the development of our knowledge of things or of the education of the senses, percepts may best be grouped according to their clearness, detail and number of connections with images and other percepts. Thus the vague, coarse and isolated percept of its mother's face which an infant has would be put in one group; the percept of the same face which the child will feel in a year or two would be put in a second group; while the exact definition and complete detail of the percept of the same face felt by a friend who was painting the mother's portrait would be put in a third class.

Percepts might also be classified as single or collective. The sight of a pencil or the sound of a tone are examples of the former; the sight of a forest or an army or the sound of a melody or of a pattering of rain are examples of the latter.

The Constitution of Percepts.—Elementary sensations are said to combine to form percepts. When the combination is by the juxtaposition in space of the elements, as when different bits of blue make a blue surface or different bits of pressure give the feeling of a hand pressed against the brow, the combination is called *colligation*. When the elements do not each exclude the other from occupying the same space, as when different tones combine to form a chord, or when tastes and smells and touch combine to form the total 'taste' of celery, the combination is called *fusion*. This combination is really a combination, not of feelings, but of the processes in the brain upon which they depend.

Exercises

1. Give illustrations of illusions and of hallucinations from your own and from your friends' experiences.

2. a. Which senses provide percepts of the form of objects?
   b. Which senses provide percepts of the texture of objects?
   c. Which senses provide percepts of the weight of objects?

3. What terms in grammar refer respectively to single and collective percepts?

4. Give three illustrations of the influence of training in replacing vague and coarse percepts by definite and detailed percepts.

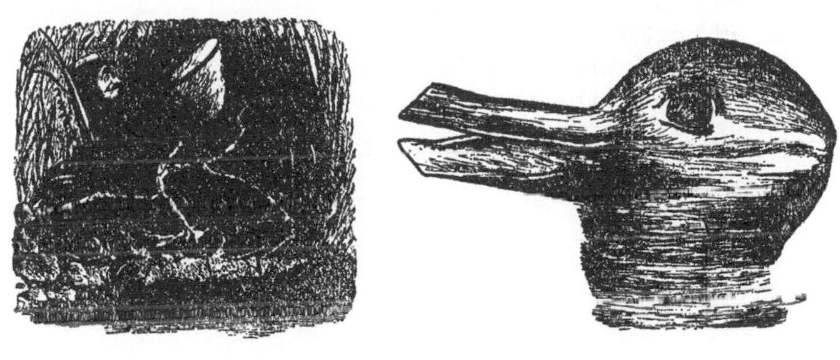

A FIG. 1 B

5. What paragraphs in the text bring out the facts stated in these quotations? For a. see § 6; for b. and c. see § 8.
   a. "Consciousness is never composed of a single sensation." (Titchener).
   b. "The consciousness of particular material things present to sense is nowadays called perception." (James).
   c. "Every perception is an acquired perception." (James).

Experiment 5. Sensations and Percepts.—a. Look at Fig. 1 A. Find the two frogs. Notice the change from a vague blur of lines to a definite picture as the frogs spring into view.

b. Look at a landscape with the head turned upside down; then with the head in its usual position.

c. Look through the pages of an illustrated magazine, held

upside down or turned through an angle of 135 degrees from its usual position. When a picture appears as a mere chaos of sensations, turn the magazine to its usual position and note the difference in the picture's definiteness and *'thingness.'*

Experiment 6. Percept and Stimulus.—Look at Fig. 1 B. What is it? Continue looking until you find another animal shown. Show the figure to six or eight people, letting each one tell at once what it is. What sentence in the text (page 36) do the results illustrate?

References

A. James, *Briefer Course,* XX. (312-315).
Stout, *Manual,* 312-391.
Titchener, *Outline,* §§ 43-51.
Angell, *Psychology,* VI., VII.

B. Ebbinghaus, *Grundzüge,* §§ 37-41.
James, *Principles,* XIX. (76-82).
Wundt, *Physiologische Psychologie,* XII.-XV.

[1] I am indebted to the publishers of St. Nicholas for permission to use Fig. 1 A.

CHAPTER III

Feelings of Things as Absent: Images and Memories

§ 9. *Mental Images*

Definition and Classification.—The term *Imagery* or *Images* is often restricted to feelings of *things* as not present. A more useful meaning and one that prevails in recent books on psychology, is *feelings of things, qualities and conditions of all sorts as not present.* In this sense of the word there may be an image to correspond to every sensation, percept, impulse or emotion. There may be images of fatigue, fear, lonesomeness and tickling, as well as of faces or tunes. The most frequent images are however of sights, sounds and movements.

Images are naturally classified according to the kind of sensation or percept or impulse or emotion to which they correspond. The most important groups are:

Images of sights:—Visual Images.
Images of sounds:—Auditory or Audile Images.
Images of feelings of movement:—Motor or Motile Images.
Images of touches:—Tactile Images.
Images of tastes:—Gustatory Images.
Images of smells:—Olfactory Images.

The readers may be unable to get images of all these different kinds. Images of tastes and of smells are comparatively rare and some individuals can be found who apparently lack visual and auditory images.

A group of images which is of much practical importance is formed by images of *words.* More of human thinking, especially of that of educated men and women, is done by imaged words than by imaged objects. It should be noted that whereas for images of objects the order of frequency is visual, auditory, motor, the order of frequency for images of words is probably *motor auditory, visual.* Possibly *auditory, motor, visual* is the order, but common opinion often mistakes a motor for an auditory image. The more one observes his images of words, the more he will find motor factors and approach agreement with the following statement by Bain:

'When we recall the impression of a word or sentence, if we do not speak it out, we feel the twitter of the organs just about to come to that point. The articulating parts —the larynx, the tongue, the lips—are all sensibly excited; a suppressed articulation is in fact the material of our recollection, the intellectual manifestation, the idea of speech.'[1]

Generic Images.—In certain cases the conditions are especially favorable for the production of vague, hazy, incomplete images; namely, when many things alike in certain features and unlike in others have been experienced. For instance, the many different percepts that have been associated with the word dog result in a tendency of the process of reproduction toward an image of a dog of indefinite and fleeting size, color and shape. In such cases the different percepts contribute elements which in some cases agree enough to reinforce each other, in others are so contradictory as to annihilate each other, and in all cases tend somewhat to give way in succession to each other. We may compare the process to that of making composite photographs in which each of a hun-

[1] Quoted by James, *Principles of Psychology,* vol. II., p. 64.

dred or so faces has its share. Or the process may be likened to the clamor of a thousand men saying something alike in part and different in other parts. Out of it all comes to the listener a vague feeling of the general thought of the assembly. A mental image which possesses clearly only the commonest features of a class of objects, being incomplete and hazy and changing in all minor details, is called a *Generic Image.*

"In dreams, one sees houses, trees and other objects, which are perfectly recognisable as such, but which remind one of the actual objects as seen 'out of the corner of the eye,' or of the pictures thrown by a badly-focused magic lantern. A man addresses us who is like a figure seen by twilight; or we travel through countries where every feature of the scenery is vague; the outlines of the hills are ill-marked, and the rivers have no defined banks. They are, in short, generic ideas of many past impressions of men, hills, and rivers. An anatomist who occupies himself intently with the examination of several specimens of some new kind of animal, in course of time acquires so vivid a conception of its form and structure, that the idea may take visible shape and become a sort of waking dream. But the figure which thus presents itself is generic, not specific. It is no copy of any one specimen, but, more or less, a mean of the series."[1]

Variation in Images.—Images differ greatly in clearness, in fidelity and in susceptibility to control. One may have a perfect distinct image of his father's face, one which accurately corresponds detail for detail with the real percept and which can be gotten at any time and retained before the mind's eye at will; but his image of a certain house or of a regular polygon of twenty sides may be vague, rough and fleeting. Between individuals the difference is even more marked. One may be able at will to feel 'before his mind's nose' the odor of roast

[1] Huxley's *'Hume,'* p. 113.

beef as a clear exact correspondent of the real sensation. Another may be utterly unable to feel it at all unless it is there. The following cases illustrate extreme cases of imagery of various sorts:—

(1) "This morning's breakfast-table is both dim and bright; it is dim if I try to think of it when my eyes are open upon any object; it is perfectly clear and bright if I think of it with my eyes closed.......All the objects are clear at once, yet when I confine my attention to any one object it becomes far more distinct........I have more power to recall color than any other one thing; if, for example, I were to recall a plate decorated with flowers, I could reproduce in a drawing the exact tone, etc. The color of anything that was on the table was perfectly vivid.—There is very little limitation to the extent of my images: I can see all four sides of a room, I can see all four sides of two, three, four, even more rooms with such distinctness that if you should ask me what was in any particular place in any one, or ask me to count the chairs, etc., I could do it without the least hesitation.—The more I learn by heart, the more clearly do I see images of my pages. Even before I can recite the lines, I can see them so that I could give them very slowly word for word, but my mind is so occupied in looking at my printed image that I have no idea of what I am saying, of the sense of it, etc. When I first found myself doing this, I used to think it was merely because I knew the lines imperfectly; but I have quite convinced myself that I really do see an image. The strongest proof that such is really the fact is I think, the following:

"I can look down the mentally seen page and see the words that *commence* all the lines, and from any one of these words I can continue the line. I find this much easier to do if the words begin in a straight line than if there are breaks."[1]

(2) "I am unable to form in my mind's eye any visual likeness of the table whatever. After many trials I can only get a hazy surface, with nothing on it or about

[1]James, *Principles of Psychology,* vol. II., p. 56.

it. I can see no variety in color, and no positive limitations in extent, while I cannot see what I see well enough to determine its position in respect to my eye, or to endow it with any quality of size. I am in the same position as to the word *dog*. I cannot see it in my mind's eye at all; and so cannot tell whether I should have to run my eye along it, if I did see it."[1]

(3) "Imagination also takes the auditory form. 'When I write a scene,' said Legouvé to Scribe, 'I *hear;* but you *see*. In each phrase which I write, the voice of the personage strikes my ear. *Vous, qui êtes le théâtre même,* your actors walk, gesticulate before your eyes; I am a *listener,* you a *spectator*'........'Nothing more true,' said Scribe. 'Do you know where I am when I write a piece? In the middle of the parterre.'[1]

(4) "If I wish to imagine that I am walking, I have to combine feelings in the parts of the body concerned in walking. This feeling is in my case most vivid in the upper part of the thigh. For every step, which I wish to imagine, I have to revive expressly such a feeling in the upper part of the thigh, just as if I wished to really move it forward, to make a real step."......

"If I try to call up in memory the walking movement of another person, say of a soldier marching, and in such wise as to imagine him first in one position (for instance with both legs on the ground and then as lifting his leg at the order *March* and putting it forward so as to take a step), I notice that I am thinking of the upper part of one of my own thighs.

"If I wish to imagine him lifting his left leg, I am aware of something in the upper part of my left thigh; if I seek to imagine him as lifting his right leg, the feeling passes back to my right thigh."......

"My memories of the movements of all inanimate objects are for the most part connected with feelings in the eye muscles. If I wish to represent to myself the motion of the clouds, I have to add the feeling of my eyes following the clouds. If I try to suppress this feel-

[1] James, *Principles of Psychology,* vol. II., pp. 57-60.

ing, the image of the movement is at once inhibited, the clouds seem unable to move. The case is the same with my images of the flight of a bird, of smoke rising, of a wagon passing by.

"I cannot imagine the sound *b* without feelings in my lips. No more can I call up the feeling in my lips of *b* without thinking of the sound."[1]

(5) "Auditory Mental Imagery. I find the auditory mental imagery in my case to be almost as important a factor in my mental life as is the visual, being a mental reproduction of the sounds I have heard—musical or otherwise. They are comparable with real sounds, not so much in intensity, but perfectly in timbre, pitch and duration. I can estimate a minute with much greater exactness mentally if I listen to the auditory mental imagery of a piece of music which takes about a minute to perform.

"The auditory mental imagery, I would say, includes all the actual word thinking that I do, which is almost always done by means of writing.

"Olfactory Mental Imagery. These are in my own case extremely numerous, probably because to me so many things have a smell, often a distinctive smell..... These mental images have to me, like those of the other senses, quite distinctive qualities. The mental image of the smell of new-mown hay is totally unlike, even as a purely mental occurrence, that of the aroma of forest leaf-mold. And the words 'tea' and 'coffee' are represented in my mind by two mental images, totally unlike."[2]

Types of Imagination.—Individuals may often be classified under types according to the kind of imagery which predominates in their streams of thought. Thus Dr. Stricker, the author of the fourth quotation given above, would be put under the motor type, while the author of the first quotation would be called a visualizer.

[1] S. Stricker, *Bewegungsvorstellungen,* pp. 12-14, and *Sprachvorstellungen,* pp. 9-10.

[2] Wilfrid Lay, *Mental Imagery,* pp. 36-37.

So would Dr. Lay, who found that 2,500 recorded mental images of his own were distributed as follows:

	Per Cent.		*Per Cent.*		*Per Cent.*
Visual	57.4	Gustatory	.6	Organic	1.1
Auditory	28.8	Thermal	2.0	Motor	.3
Olfactory	5.9	Tactile	3.8	Emotional	.1

The majority of individuals do not, however, show so emphatic a predominance of one kind of imagery as to be put surely in any one class. They are mixed types. For instance the reader will probably find that he or she has visual images most frequently, auditory next and motor next, as do the majority; that in his class or among his friends cases of the almost exclusive use of any one kind of imagery are rare.

Image and Percept.—The image, as defined, is never the exact duplicate of the sensation or percept to which it corresponds. If it were, one would feel the thing as present and act as if it were. Indeed the most useful characteristic of an image is that it does *not* duplicate the sensation or percept. Otherwise we should all be like sleep-walkers and madmen, confusing fact with fancy in the most absurd and dangerous ways.

Images, like percepts, are the result of a process of acquisition. At the start of life we have neither, and for some time the two are confused,—at least in memory, as is witnessed by the innocent lies of three year olds who tell of lions running down the street and of dogs as big as houses or as small as mice.

Productive Imagination.—So far only those images have been described which at least roughly correspond to real things and conditions. There also occur images which correspond to nothing real, but are new combinations. One can picture a beast with an elephant's head, a lion's body and a giraffe's legs. There is in these cases a correspondence not of the total image with some real thing, but only of parts of the image with parts or elements of real things. In our fancies and dreams we thus make the most extraordinary and elaborate combinations of the old familiar elements. The names (1) *Reproductive Imagination* and (2) *Productive Imagination* are used for (1) the capacity of getting images that repeat whole things experienced and (2) the capacity of getting images of things never experienced on a basis of old elements and parts.

The capacity to thus create a new world from the ruins of past experiences is one of the primary sources of human achievement. When directed by wise insight it becomes a part of the creative genius of poets, inventors and men of science. On the basis of the same experiences one man imagines the steam engine, another man nothing; out of the same stuff one man creates a tawdry play of revenge, another a Hamlet.

§ 10. *Memories*

Definitions.—In the common usage of language the words memory and to remember refer to four distinct things:—

(1) The presence of mental images; *e.g.*, 'Can you remember his face?' usually means, 'Can you call up a visual image of his face?'

(2) The feeling of a thing as having been experienced; *e.g.*, 'I remember your face but I cannot place it.' Recognition is a better name for this sort of feeling.

(3) The feeling of a thing or event as belonging to some definite experience of one's own in the past, or, in the words of Professor James, "Knowledge of an event, or fact, of which meantime we have not been thinking,

with the additional consciousness that we have thought or experienced it before;" *e.g.*, 'Do you remember how you fell from your horse here last summer?' means, 'Can you call to mind the event, and feel that you experienced it?'

(4) The continued existence of connections that have been formed between ideas or feelings and acts or acts and acts; *e.g.*, 'Do you remember your Latin?', 'Do you remember how to write shorthand?', and 'Do you remember how to throw an out curve?' refer to the presence not of feelings of things past but of connections made in the past. Permanence of connections or associations is a better name for these facts.

Memory Proper.—The word memory, or rather memories, may best be kept rather strictly for the feelings of class (3) of the above. Such feelings are evidently complex. They involve far more than the mere repetition of a feeling. Like images they are feelings of a thing or event as not present. They also involve the perception of time, since they are feelings of things or events as having been present in the past The consciousness of self enters, also, since they are feelings of a thing or event as having been in one's own past experience. Like judgments they imply an affirmation that such a state of affairs is (here was) the case. It would indeed not be unfair to define memories (meaning by the word class (3) above) as *judgments concerning one's own past experience.*

The facts about the permanence of connections will be presented in Part III, since they are explainable by the laws of the mind's action,—belong, that is, to dynamic psychology. Why different individuals possess different degrees of ability in retaining connections once formed, what decides whether one shall be able to call up a given fact or not, how connections may most readily be made permanent,—are samples of the questions that will arise.

Exercises

1. Study carefully the picture your mind calls up of your breakfast-table of this morning as Galton directs in his 'Questions on Visualizing' and then write down your answers to the first three questions of his list. Where would you class yourself in visual imagery and in color representation, using Galton's scale (printed on page 55 f.)?

2. Make the observations and answer the questions as directed by Galton, so far as you have time. What kinds of images do you lack entirely? What kinds are little developed? What kinds are most prominent? Compare your answers with those of three or four of your friends.

In answering the questions one must beware of:—

(1) Confusing the image of the name of a thing with the image of the thing itself. That I can call up the word *bitter* does not mean that I can have an image of a bitter taste.

(2) Confusing the fact that one can act as if a feeling were present in his mind with the fact of the real presence of the feeling. The same act may have various antecedents. That I can draw my finger around an oblong space in the air does not imply that I can have a visual image of an oblong. That I shiver when someone is hurt does not imply that I feel an image of pain.

(3) Confusing the knowledge that something happened with an image of its happening. That I can now feel that I was angry does not mean that I feel a mental image of the emotion, anger.

(4) Confusing the process of arousing certain conditions and so having a certain real feeling, with the process of arousing an image of that feeling. That I can, by thinking of certain events, get a feeling of anger, does not mean that I can get an image of the feeling of anger. That by calling up thoughts of the country I can arouse a feeling of desire does not mean that I can feel an image of the feeling of desire.

Galton's 'Questions on Visualizing and Other Allied Faculties'

"The object of these Questions is to elicit the degree in which different persons possess the power of seeing images in their mind's eye, and of reviving past sensations.

From inquiries I have already made, it appears that remarkable variations exist both in the strength and in the quality of these faculties, and it is highly probable that a statistical inquiry into them will throw light upon more than one psychological problem.

Before addressing yourself to any of the Questions . . . . think of some definite object—suppose it is your breakfast-table as you sat down to it this morning—and consider carefully the picture that rises before your mind's eye.

1. *Illumination.*—Is the image dim or fairly clear? Is its brightness comparable to that of the actual scene?

2. *Definition.*—Are all the objects pretty well defined at the same time, or is the place of sharpest definition at any one moment more contracted than it is in a real scene?

3. *Colouring.*—Are the colours of the china, of the toast, bread crust, mustard, meat, parsley, or whatever may have been on the table, quite distinct and natural?

4. *Extent of field of view.*—Call up the image of some panoramic view (the walls of your room might suffice). Can you force yourself to see mentally a wider range of it than could be taken in by any single glance of the eyes? Can you mentally see more than three faces of a die, or more than one hemisphere of a globe at the same instant of time?

5. *Distance of images.*—Where do mental images appear to be situated? Within the head, within the eye-ball, just in front of the eyes, or at a distance corresponding to reality? Can you project an image upon a piece of paper?

6. *Command over images.*—Can you retain a mental picture steadily before the eyes? When you do so, does it grow brighter or dimmer? When the act of retaining it becomes wearisome, in what part of the head or eye-ball is the fatigue felt?

7. *Persons.*—Can you recall with distinctness the features of all near relations and many other persons? Can you at will cause your mental image of any or most of them to sit, stand, or turn slowly round? Can you deliberately seat the image of a well-known person in a chair and see it with enough distinctness

to enable you to sketch it leisurely (supposing yourself able to draw)?

8. *Scenery.*—Do you preserve the recollection of scenery with much precision of detail, and do you find pleasure in dwelling on it? Can you easily form mental pictures from the descriptions of scenery that are so frequently met with in novels and books of travel?

9. *Comparison with reality.*—What difference do you perceive between a very vivid mental picture called up in the dark, and a real scene? Have you ever mistaken a mental image for a reality when in health and wide awake?

10. *Numerals and dates.*—Are these invariably associated in your mind with any peculiar mental imagery, whether of written or printed figures, diagrams, or colours? If so, explain fully, and say if you can account for the association.

11. *Specialties.*—If you happen to have special aptitudes for mechanics, mathematics (either geometry of three dimensions or pure analysis), mental arithmetic, or chess-playing blindfold, please explain fully how far your processes depend on the use of visual images, and how far otherwise?

12. Call up before your imagination the objects specified in the six following paragraphs, numbered A to F, and consider carefully whether your mental representation of them generally, is in each group very faint, faint, fair, good, or vivid and comparable to the actual sensation:—

A. *Light and colour.*—An evenly clouded sky (omitting all landscape), first bright, then gloomy. A thick surrounding haze, first white, then successively blue, yellow, green, and red.

B. *Sound.*—The beat of rain against the window panes, the crack of a whip, a church bell, the hum of bees, the whistle of a railway, the clinking of tea-spoons and saucers, the slam of a door.

C. *Smells.*—Tar, roses, an oil-lamp blown out, hay, violets, a fur coat, gas, tobacco.

D. *Tastes.*—Salt, sugar, lemon juice, raisins, chocolate, currant jelly.

E. *Touch.*—Velvet, silk, soap, gum, sand, dough, a crisp dead leaf, the prick of a pin.

F. *Other sensations.*—Heat, hunger, cold, thirst, fatigue, fever, drowsiness, a bad cold.

13. *Music.*—Have you any aptitude for mentally recalling music, or for imagining it?

14. *At different ages.*—Do you recollect what your powers of visualizing, etc., were in childhood? Have they varied much within your recollection?" (F. Galton, *Inquiries Into Human Faculty,* pp. 378-380.)

GALTON'S SCALE OF VIVIDNESS AND FIDELITY IN VISUAL IMAGERY

"Highest.—Brilliant, distinct, never blotchy.

First Suboctile.—The image once seen is perfectly clear and bright.

First Octile.—I can see my breakfast-table or any equally familiar thing with my mind's eye quite as well in all particulars as I can do if the reality is before me.

First Quartile.—Fairly clear; illumination of actual scene is fairly represented. Well defined. Parts do not obtrude themselves, but attention has to be directed to different points in succession to call up the whole.

Middlemost.—Fairly clear. Brightness probably at least from one-half to two-thirds of the original. Definition varies very much, one or two objects being much more distinct than the others, but the latter come out clearly if attention be paid to them.

Last Quartile.—Dim, certainly not comparable to the actual scene. I have to think separately of the several things on the table to bring them clearly before the mind's eye, and when I think of some things the others fade away in confusion.

Last Octile.—Dim and not comparable in brightness to the real scene. Badly defined with blotches of light; very incomplete; very little of one object is seen at one time.

Last Suboctile.—I am very rarely able to recall any object whatever with any sort of distinctness. Very occasionally an object or image will recall itself, but even then it is more like a generalised image than an individual one. I seem to be almost destitute of visualising power as under control.

Lowest.—My powers are zero. To my consciousness there is almost no association of memory with objective visual impressions. I recollect the table, but do not see it.

IN COLOUR REPRESENTATION

Highest.—Perfectly distinct, bright and natural.

First Suboctile.—White cloth, blue china, argand coffee-pot, buff stand with sienna drawing, toast—all clear.

First Octile.—All details seen perfectly.

First Quartile.—Colours distinct and natural till I begin to puzzle over them.

Middlemost.—Fairly distinct, though not certain that they are accurately recalled.

Last Quartile.—Natural, but very indistinct.

Last Octile.—Faint; can only recall colours by a special effort for each.

Last Suboctile.—Power is nil.

Lowest.—Power is nil." (*Inquiries Into Human Faculty,* pp. 93-94.)

First suboctile means the ability exceeded by one sixteenth of people; first octile means the ability exceeded by one eighth; first quartile means the ability exceeded by one fourth; last quartile means the ability exceeded by three fourths; last octile means the ability exceeded by seven eighths, last suboctile means the ability exceeded by fifteen sixteenths.

3. Compare the imagery of the author of the following statement with that of the individuals quoted in § 9.

"When I seek to represent a row of soldiers marching, all I catch is a view of stationary legs first in one phase of movement and then in another, and these views are extremely imperfect and momentary. Occasionally (especially when I try to stimulate my imagination as by repeating Victor Hugo's lines about the regiment,

'Leur pas est si correct, sans tarder ni courir,
Qu'on croit voir des ciseaux se fermer et s'ouvrir,')

I seem to get an instantaneous glimpse of an actual movement, but it is to the last degree dim and uncertain. All these images seem at first to be purely retinal. I think, however, that rapid eye-movements accompany them, though these latter give rise to such slight feelings that they are almost impossible of detection. Absolutely no leg-movements of my own are there; in fact, to call such up arrests my imagination of the soldiers. My optical images are in general very dim, dark, fugitive and contracted. It would be utterly impossible to *draw* from them, and yet I perfectly well distinguish one from the other. My auditory images are excessively inadequate reproductions of their originals. I have *no* images of taste or smell. Touch-imagination is fairly distinct, but comes very little into play with most objects thought of. Neither is all my thought verbalized; for I have shadowy schemes of relation, as apt to terminate in a nod of the head or an expulsion of the breath as in a definite word. On the whole, vague images or sensations of movement inside of my head towards the various parts of space in which the terms I am thinking of either lie or are momentarily symbolized to lie together with movements of the breath through my pharynx and nostrils, form a by no means inconsiderable part of my *thought-stuff.*" (James, *Principles of Psychology,* vol. II., p. 65.)

Experiment 7. After Images and Recalled Images.—Cut out of a sheet of black paper, say 10 inches square, a cross with arms each an inch wide and two inches long. Fasten the sheet against the glass of a window so that a bright light comes through the cross shaped opening. Sitting at a distance of six or eight feet, look steadily at the center of the cross for a minute and a half or longer. Then look at a white screen (for instance a sheet or towel hung against the wall) A duplicate of the cross, but dark with a light background will be seen. How does this so-called *after image* differ from the visual image you call up in memory of a dark cross on a light background:—(a) in persistence, (b) in seeming a real object, (c) in location, (d) in modification by your will, (e) in intensity?

References

A. James, *Briefer Course,* XVIII. (287-288), XIX.
Stout, *Manual,* 393-417, 435-446.
Titchener, *Outline,* §§ 70-80.
Angell, *Psychology,* VIII., IX.

B. Ebbinghaus, *Grundzüge,* §§ 48-50.
James, *Principles,* XVI. (643-652), XVIII.
Wundt, *Physiologische Psychologie,* XVIII. (§ 3), XIX. (§ 6).

CHAPTER IV

Feelings of Facts: Feelings of Relationships, Meanings and Judgments

§ 11. *Feelings of Relationships*

Contrasted with Feelings of Things and Qualities.—As you look at this page you are conscious not only of the words, 'Feelings of Relationships,' but also of the fact that these words are at the top of this page; you feel, that is, the *'aboveness'* of these words. As you think of this chapter you are aware also that it is a part of the whole book; you feel, that is, its relationship to the whole. You feel, too, the unlikeness of the black letters to the white page. As you read in the first sentence the *not only,* you feel the incompleteness of the idea immediately to come; and as you read the *but also,* you feel the belonging-together-ness or to-be-added-to-ness of the next coming idea with the idea, 'percepts of words.'

We may thus feel things and qualities and conditions, not as mere bare existences, but as related in space and time,—as more than, less than, equal to, part of, whole containing, like, unlike, opposite to, derived from, superior to or inferior to some other fact. Amongst parts of speech, prepositions and conjunctions express feelings, not of things or qualities, but of relationships. There are feelings of in-ness, beside-ness, beyond-ness, with-ness, if-ness, but-ness and although-ness as truly as of the sun or moon, of black or white, of fatigue or pleasure.

These feelings are among the commonest features of mental life. Witness how much disappears from any statement,—*e.g.*, the preamble to the United States Constitution,—when words expressing feelings of relationship are omitted from the text.

"We the people the States form perfect, establish justice, insure domestic tranquillity, the defense, the welfare, the blessings liberty ourselves posterity do ordain establish this Constitution States America."[1]

Their Attributes.—It is hard to describe feelings of relationships. Anyone knows that when he thinks, 'He is sick: *nevertheless,*' he feels a different expectation toward the coming thought than if he heard or thought, 'He is sick, *therefore.*' But it would be impossible to describe the feeling to one who had not felt it himself and it would take rather long statement to describe it to oneself. Two characteristics feelings of relationships almost invariably possess. In the first place they are fleeting, evanescent, intangible mental states. No sooner does one try to examine them than they are gone. One can keep the same percept in mind for some time; can hold the same image constant for at least a number of seconds. But one rarely thinks neverthelessness or but-ness or above-ness for any appreciable time. Feelings of relationship are among those transitory states of mind which Professor James calls the *fringes* of thought; they are the almost unseen web of connections in which are set the obvious percepts and images and the somewhat less obvious feelings of meaning. In the second place they almost invariably occur, not by themselves alone but in a context either as ele-

[1] Some of the words retained are relational if we consider their real meaning. Form and establish, ordain and secure may thus be held to express a feeling of causing; domestic and posterity to express feelings of unlikeness.

ments of complex mental states,—'fringes' or 'tendencies' of percepts and images, or as transitive, intermediate feelings, joining two mental states. We feel, not *more* alone but *more than some given thing;* not merely *and* but *John and James.* We feel things as relative or as related rather than things and relations.[1] To supplement this account of the nature of these elusive feelings, I quote from Professor William James, who first emphasized their importance.

"If there be such things as feelings at all, *then so surely as relations between objects exist in rerum natura, so surely, and more surely, do feelings exist to which these relations are known.* There is not a conjunction or a preposition, and hardly an adverbial phrase, syntactic form, or inflection of voice, in human speech, that does not express some shading or other of relation which we at some moment actually feel to exist between the larger objects of our thought........

We ought to say a feeling of *and,* a feeling of *if,* a feeling of *but* and a feeling of *by,* quite as readily as we say a feeling of *blue* or a feeling of *cold.*"

"When we read such phrases as 'naught but,' 'either one or the other,' 'a is b,' 'but,' 'although it is, nevertheless,' 'it is an excluded middle, there is no *tertium quid,*' and a host of other verbal skeletons of logical relation, is it true that there is nothing more in our minds than the words themselves as they pass? What then is the meaning of the words which we think we understand as we read? What makes that meaning different in one phrase from what it is in the other? 'Who?' 'When?' 'Where?' Is the difference of felt meaning in these interrogatives nothing more than their difference of sound? And is it

[1]Occasionally perhaps the pure feeling of a relationship holds the field by itself. The mere feeling of unity or of difference seems to enthrall us without our being able to say *what* is thus unified or similar. The following sentence, *e. g.*, seems to represent nothing more than jumbled feelings of relationship. "There are no differences but differences of degree between different degrees of difference and no difference."

not (just like the difference of a sound itself) known and understood in an affection of consciousness correlative to it, though so impalpable to direct examination? Is not the same true of such negatives as 'no,' 'never,' 'not yet?'

The truth is that large tracts of human speech are nothing but *signs of direction* in thought, of which direction we nevertheless have an acutely discriminative sense, though no definite sensorial image plays any part in it whatsoever. Sensorial images are stable psychic facts; we can hold them still and look at them as long as we like. These bare images of logical movement, on the contrary, are psychic transitions, always on the wing, so to speak, and not to be glimpsed except in flight. Their function is to lead from one set of images to another. As they pass, we feel both the waxing and the waning images in a way altogether peculiar and a way quite different from the way of their full presence."

"Every definite image in the mind is steeped and dyed in the free water that flows around it. With it goes the sense of its relations, near and remote, the dying echo of whence it came to us, the dawning sense of whither it is to lead. The significance, the value, of the image is all in this halo or penumbra that surrounds and escorts it,—or rather that is fused into one with it and has become bone of its bone and flesh of its flesh; leaving it, it is true, an image of the same *thing* it was before, but making it an image of that thing newly taken and freshly understood."[1]

Classification.—The more important feelings of relationship may be classified as follows:—

Feelings of Objective Relationships—

Of Relationships of Space.
" " " Time.
" " " Substance and Quality.

Feelings of Logical or Intellectual or Subjective Relationships—

[1] James, *Principles of Psychology,* vol. I., pp. 245-255 passim.

Of Relationships of Identity.
" " " Equality.
" " " Likeness.
" " " Unlikeness.
" " " Opposition.
" " " Part and Whole.
" " " Cause and Effect.
" " " Condition and Result.
" " " Concession.

Feelings of Relationships and Logical Thought.—Feelings of Relationships are essential features of logical thinking. Especially important for it are feelings of the intellectual relationships, such as likeness and difference, and cause and effect. Compare, for instance, the paragraph A, which requires no thought and which leads mainly to a series of images in a scholar's mind, with the paragraph B, which involves thought and leads to real comprehension. Count the number of words standing for relationships in each.

A.

The Nile overflows annually. The land in Egypt is fertile. The soil of the hills to the south is rich. The river deposits the soil. The land produces great crops of wheat. The river plains of China produce large crops of rice. Egypt used to be called the granary of Rome. The method of cultivation in Egypt is by hand labor. The people are uninventive. The people are uneducated.

B.

Because of the annual overflow of the Nile the land in Egypt is fertilized by a deposit of rich soil brought down from the hills to the south. The land thus produces great crops of wheat for the same reason that the river plains of China produce large crops of rice. Hence Egypt used to be called the granary of Rome. The inferior methods of cultivation, largely by hard labor, are due to the lack of inventiveness and of education among the population who sow by hand.

The dependence of logical thinking or reasoning upon feelings of relationships is shown also by a comparison of studies like grammar or geometry, which are conspicuously rational, with one like spelling, ability in which is consistent with almost all degrees of reasoning power. Grammar bristles with relationships of subject, object, modifier and modified, dependent and independent, actor and acted upon, condition, concession and the like. Geometry is practically a series of propositions based on the relationships of identity, equality, greater than and less than. Spelling, however, is chiefly a matter of clear, accurate percepts of words and permanent associations of their images with the sounds and meanings of the words. Only occasionally are there words whose spelling is to be inferred from their likeness to others or from their being wholes, the parts of which are known.

The Development of Feelings of Relationships.— Feelings of relationships develop later in childhood than feelings of things and qualities; *e.g.*, conjunctions are among the latest words learned, and complex sentences involving the expression, in clauses, of feelings of condition, cause, opposition, and the like, appear much later than simple sentences. Children asked to give the word meaning the opposite of a given word, to give the word meaning just what the given word does not mean, will answer correctly and quickly in the case of words like *day, work, rich, empty,* or *to hate,* at an age when they would answer only partially and slowly in the case of *with, different, more* or *part,* and would in most cases fail utterly with *and, because* or *if*. The feelings of space- and time-relationships are felt much earlier than the so-called logical relationships such as cause, condition or concession.

The ease with which feelings of relationships, especially of relationships other than those of space and time, are acquired and the extent to which they are used by any individual, are in direct ratio to his intellectual capacity. The brighter the child, the more they will be in evidence. Very weak minded children never come to feel them.

Exercises

1. Make a list of ten or more words expressing feelings of relationships other than those of time and space.

2. Give instances of other parts of speech than conjunctions and prepositions which may express feelings of relationships.

3. Of the following, which depends the more on feelings of relationship: (a) ability in computation or (b) ability in doing arithmetical problems?

4. Answer the same question in the case of (a) knowledge of syntax and (b) knowledge of vocabularies.

5. Name parts of speech that never express feelings of relationships.

6. Pick out the words or phrases expressing feelings of relationship contained in the two quotations below. Which quotation has the more words expressing intellectual relationships?

......"At the helm
A seeming mermaid steers: the silken tackle
Swell with the touches of those flower-soft hands,
That yarely frame the office. From the barge
A strange invisible perfume hits the sense
Of the adjacent wharfs. The city cast
Her people out upon her; and Antony,
Enthroned i' the market-place, did sit alone,
Whistling to the air; which, but for vacancy,
Had gone to gaze on Cleopatra too.
And made a gap in nature."

Antony and Cleopatra; Act II, Scene II.

"What is the task which philosophers set themselves to perform; and why do they philosophize at all? Almost every one will immediately reply: They desire to attain a conception of the frame of things which shall on the whole be more rational than that somewhat chaotic view which every one by nature carries about with him under his hat. But suppose this rational conception attained, how is the philosopher to recognize it for what it is, and not let it slip through ignorance? The only answer can be that he will recognize its rationality as he recognizes everything else, by certain subjective marks with which it affects him. When he gets the marks, he may know that he has got the rationality." (W. James, *The Will to Believe,* p. 63.)

7. Copy the first page of this text book omitting all words that express and arouse feelings of relationships. Observe the result.

8. Make up intelligible sentences which, like the example below, shall be composed in the main of words expressing feelings of neither things nor emotions nor sensible qualities nor feelings meaning such, but only of relationships. "Although ——— is not a product and ——— cannot be equal to a derivative still the addition on the one hand and the subtraction on the other of necessity counteract each other. The total result therefore may be just the same as it was in the previous process." The only words here which in order to make sense need be the names of things are the two to be supplied in the blank spaces.

9. Try to express the law of gravitation or any theorem in geometry, or to explain the change of the seasons, without using words that express and arouse feelings of relationships. Try to express, subject to the same limitation, the experiences of an hour in a storm. Why is the second task easy of accomplishment and the first so hard?

§ 12. *Feelings of Meaning*

Their Nature and Attributes.—Sensations, percepts, images and emotions are *direct* feelings of things, qualities and conditions. The feeling appears to *be* the thing. But we can feel that we mean or refer to a thing without directly feeling *it.* Thus one can think of or mean or refer in thought to his father without at the time seeing him or having a mental image of his appearance. That this power of meaning objects, in addition to and apart from feeling them as present or as absent, exists, can be proved by examining one's thoughts and also by the fact that we can mean or refer to objects, perceptions or images of which are impossible. For instance you can *think of,* though you cannot see or imagine, ten million pine trees growing in one row, or a line one millionth of an inch long, or a thousand angels all standing on one pin head, or Romulus and Remus, or King Alfred of England, or a flying machine without wings or balloons. Furthermore a dozen men may each have a similar feeling of meaning although the sensed and imaged parts of their thoughts are to the last degree dissimilar. Thus though one man hears 'Cinq et cinq font dix,' another 'Fünf und fünf sind zehn,' and a third, 'Five and five are ten;' though the first man has a visual image of $5+5=10$, the second a motor image of the incipient movements of saying 'Fünf und fünf sind zehn,' and the third no image at all, yet the feeling of the *meaning* may be the same in each case.

The bulk of our thinking is in fact not concerned with direct feelings of things, but with mere references to them. We can do hundreds of examples about dollars and cents and hours, about feet of carpet and pounds of sugar, with never a percept of real money or carpets and with few or no mental pictures of the sight of coins or the taste of sugar. We can argue about the climate of a country with few or no mental pictures of black skies, drenched skins, or muddy soil. It is sufficient for our purposes if we feel that the words or other symbols in which we think *stand for* or *represent* or *refer to* the real things.

The sound or sight or articulation, felt or imagined, of a word,—*i.e.,* the percept or image of it,—is the least important thing about it. The word or symbol need not be in the least like the real thing. What it refers to or stands for is the essential. Eleven dollars has a smoother, pleasanter sound than sixty-six buckets of gold shekels; the word victuals is as a word more painful than the word pain; H_2SO_4 is a rather bland and agreeable sound. Any symbol will do for any real thing. In fact the whole body of language and of scientific and mathematical symbols has for one of its chief ends to furnish us a way to mean and think of things (and also of qualities, conditions, emotions and relationships) without directly feeling or imagining them. The chief office of percepts and images of words is to be carriers of meanings.

So far I have described only feelings meaning things, but we can mean qualities, conditions, emotions, impulses or relationships as well. The reader can think, 'Red is a bright color,' without any red in his actual field of vision. He can think, 'Great fatigue overcame the mind of the general,' or, 'In his anger he smote him to the ground,' without feeling in the least tired or angry in fact or fancy. He can think, 'A strong impulse to sneeze nearly betrayed the servant's presence,' without himself being tempted to sneeze. He can think, 'The relation of condition contrary to the fact is expressed in Latin by the subjunctive,' without feeling any unfulfilled condition. Anything that we have ever felt in fact or fancy can later be meant or referred to. We can not only have or, one might say, *be* our feelings, but can at our convenience think of them through symbols devised for the purpose.

Classification.—Chief among our feelings of meaning are:—

1. Feelings that mean single facts or feelings of individual reference. Such feelings we call *Individual Notions.* Examples are our feelings of the meanings of the italicized words in the following:—

Julius Caesar is dead.
His anger was terrible to witness.
My dog is lost.

2. Feelings that mean groups or classes of facts or any one or some part of a group or class of facts. They are called *General Notions, Class Ideas, Concepts* or feelings of general reference. Examples are:—

A. Meaning a group or class.

Men are mortal.
Hospitals are useful.
Sponges are animals.
Teachers should possess tact.

B. Meaning anyone of a group or class.

Any man is sure to die.
A hospital benefits the community.
A sponge is not a plant.
A teacher needs tact.

C. Meaning some part of a group or class.

Many men die before they are forty years old.
Some hospitals are better managed than others.
Certain varieties of sponges are commercially valuable.

3. Feelings that mean some part or quality or aspect independently of the thing of which it is a part or quality or aspect. Such feelings are called *Abstract Ideas* or *Abstractions,* or feelings of reference to a quality or attribute. Examples are:—

All bodies possess *weight.*
The *heat* is intolerable.
All is lost save *honor.*

Feelings of Meaning and Images.—An individual notion may be and often is accompanied by an image more or less exact of the fact for which it stands, but in the nature of the case there can be no exact image of the fact referred to by an abstract or general notion. Of courage that is no particular act of courage, but is mere courage; of velocity which is neither fast nor slow, neither of a cannon-ball nor of a feather falling, but is mere velocity; of men that are not old or young, sick or well, white or black, with legs or without, intelligent or idiotic, but are all men; of animals that include a hundred thousand different species,—no image can be formed. Often a vague, hazy, mixed and changing image of some of the facts meant,—that is to say, a generic image,—accompanies a feeling of absolute or general meaning, but still oftener the image is not of the fact meant at all. The commonest image present is that of the *word* that is used for the fact, not of anything like the fact.

Feelings of Meaning and Reasoning.—It is largely by means of these feelings of meaning or reference that the life of real thought is carried on. Individual notions allow one to think of a fact conveniently without waiting for a percept or image of it and to keep in mind the sameness of a thing in spite of its changes. General notions present in a sort of short-hand the results of many experiences and refer to thousands of possible percepts, images and individual actions in a single word. By abstract ideas a man can break up the endless complexities of the world's objects into a comparatively small number of elements and can think the one quality which is the important subject of thought at the time without being bothered by its concrete accompaniments—can argue about courage, or industry, or subtraction, or velocity without having the mind clouded by hundreds of images of brave deeds or sums from arithmetic books, or the like. From a comparison of individual facts he can derive a general notion. From finding that an individual fact belongs to a general class about which something is true, he can assert that that thing is true of the individual fact.

Man thus comes to work over the world of actual experiences into a world of objects and relations, thought of, classified and broken up into elements. And through this world of thought he acquires new knowledge of, and enlarged control over, the world of experience. In this world of thought are the highest activities of mental life; by it are won the greatest triumphs of man over his environment.

Exercises

1. Classify the feelings of meaning aroused by reading the italicized words in the following sentences into individual notions, general notions and abstractions:—

> O, what a rogue and peasant slave am *I*.
> *He* would drown the *stage* with *tears*
> And cleave the general ear with horrid *speech,*
> Make mad *the guilty* and appall *the free.*
>
> For who would bear *the whips* and *scorns* of *time,*
> The oppressor's *wrong,* the proud man's *contumely,*
> The *pangs* of despised love, the law's delay,
> The *insolence* of office and *the spurns,*
> That *patient merit* of *the unworthy* takes.
>
> Since *my dear soul* was mistress of her choice
> And could of *men* distinguish, *her election*
> Hath sealed *thee* for *herself.*

2. Of the following studies, which two are most concerned with individual notions? Which two are most concerned with abstractions? Latin Grammar, History, Manual Training, Algebra, Chemistry.

3. Name two studies which do not deal with individual notions at all.

§ 13. *Judgments*

Definition.—In an early chapter it was stated that thoughts were rarely strings of isolated sensations, percepts, images or feelings of meaning; in the present chapter the relating, transitional, connecting feelings which help to make the complex whole thoughts of real life have been described. One important group of these complex whole thoughts comprises those which are called *Judgments.* They are feelings that a certain state of affairs is or is not the case, that a certain relationship does or does not exist between certain things. They are feelings that affirm or deny something about something,—such feelings as are ordinarily expressed in declarative sentences.[1] According to many logic books the judgment feeling is always one that relates *two* terms, and such statements as, 'The dog runs,' and 'The snow falls,' really mean, 'The dog is a running thing,' and 'The snow is a falling object.' This explanation may do no harm in logic, but it is psychologically false. One may have a judgment feeling with one term as well as with two, on the basis of a percept as well as of a comparison. The thought, 'The snow falls,' is a judgment, not that the snow is in the class a falling object, but that a certain state of affairs, 'snow falling,' is the case.

Judgments and Thought.—It is as combined in judgments that our feelings of things, conditions, qualities and relations are most influential in the intellectual life. Conversation is largely the expression of judgments. Still more so is the reading-matter of newspapers,

[1] Interrogative sentences also may express judgments plus an attitude of inquiry concerning their correspondence with reality. Thus 'Is John a tall man?' equals 'John a tall man. Is it so?' The interrogative state of mind in turn is often expressed as an outright judgment plus a query, as in the German, *'Er ist ein grosser Mann. Nicht wahr?'*

magazines and books. Every scientific formula, every mathematical equation, every philosophical principle—each is an expressed judgment. In childhood intellectual progress is marked by the transformation of mere percepts and images and vaguely felt relationships into judgments. Throughout life the thoughtful, as opposed to the sensuous or dreamy or scatter-brained, man or woman, is one whose mental states consist largely of well-defined judgments.

Classification.—Judgments may be *Individual* or *General* or *Abstract* according as they affirm or deny something about a thing or about a group of things or about an abstract quality. Judgments are called *Analytic* when they affirm or deny something about an object which was implicit in the thought of the object; *e.g.*, 'The light is bright:' 'His breathing is regular;' 'A is A.' They are called *Synthetic* when they affirm or deny something about an object which is a new contribution to the thought of the object; *e.g.*, 'The square root of 2 is 1.41421356;' 'Malaria is caused by the bite of a mosquito;' 'The most frequent age of graduation from American colleges is about 22 years and 10 months.' It should be noted that what is an analytic judgment in one case may be synthetic in another. Thus for someone who had noticed merely breathing but had not noticed varieties of breathing, 'His breathing is regular' would be a synthetic judgment. Such a person could have thought of the breathing without having its regularity implicit in the thought. 'A is A' might be a synthetic judgment in the case of a very young child.

Further classifications may be found in text books on logic. The student unacquainted with the elements of logic will do well to read Chapters I, III, VI and VIII of Aikins' *Principles of Logic,* or equivalent chapters in some similar book.

No more time need be spent with the descriptive psychology of judgments. In Part III the conditions of their development and action will concern us for many pages.

Exercises

1. Give illustrations of:—
   (a) Individual judgments.
   (b) General judgments.
   (c) Abstract judgments.
2. State also, in the case of each illustration given, whether it is an analytic or a synthetic judgment.
3. What kind of sentence does *not* express judgments?
4. Which arouses the more judgments, a story read or music heard?
5. With which are judgments most associated, learning a science like physics or learning an art like painting?

References

A. James, *Briefer Course,* XI. (160-167), XIV.
Stout, *Manual,* 447-489.
Titchener, *Outline,* §§ 82-83.
Angell, *Psychology,* X.

B. Ebbinghaus, *Grundzüge,* §§ 42-43.
James, *Principles,* IX. (245-259), XII.

CHAPTER V

FEELINGS OF PERSONAL CONDITIONS: EMOTIONS

§ 14. *The Nature of the Emotions*

Emotions Contrasted with Thoughts.—Sensations, percepts and images, and feelings of meaning, relationship and judgment agree in being connected with what in common usage is called the life of thought. They would all be put by psychologists under the head of *intellection* or *cognition.*

The emotions form in a sense a radically different group of mental facts. Love, hate, fear, jealousy, anger, joy, sorrow and the like, are feelings, not of or about things or bodily conditions recognized as such, but of one's own conditions, unreferred to bodily facts. They have, that is, a subjective or personal as opposed to an objective, reference. The emotional state of mind, in which one's own mental condition is paramount, is opposed to the intellectual state of mind, in which some object of thought is paramount. Besides possessing this subjective quality, the emotions are less subject to elaboration and manipulation than are sensations, percepts and images. They do not connect with one another so as to form any system or order as do the feelings of things, meanings and relationships. They are essentially isolated and incoherent. In the third place, we do not master them and use them at will for intellectual and practical ends as we do our ideas and judgments; rather they master us. For the time being one *is* the emotion.

Emotions and Sensations.—It is however true that between certain emotions and certain sensations no clear line of distinction can be drawn. The distinctions just made approach a vanishing point in the case of such sensations as dizziness, fatigue or nausea, and such emotions as ennui, interest, zeal, stage-fright, and the animal types of jealousy and love. Stage-fright is a feeling of as definite a thing as nausea. One can master zeal and use it to intellectual advantage rather better than nausea.

The emotions are in fact closely allied to, and perhaps are one division of, the internal sensations. Whether we shall say that the feeling of well-being is a sensation or an emotion depends upon whether we do or do not recognize it as a feeling of bodily condition, refer it to the body as we do hunger or leave it as an unreferred subjective feeling as we do ambition. One person will feel it in the one way, another in another; one person will feel it at one time as an unreferred feeling, but at another time, say after taking a medical course, will refer it definitely to his body. Indeed one theory of the nature of the emotions is that they are made up of the same stuff as sensations plus greater or less amounts of the feelings of pleasantness or unpleasantness.

§ 15. *The Classification of the Emotions*

Classifications are Arbitrary.—In our present ignorance of the differences in physiological basis of the different emotions, any method of classifying them must be largely arbitrary. Different students of the subjects consequently have widely different opinions, and in no classification can the groups be sharply separated from one another.

A classification does however serve the useful purpose of displaying the variety of the emotional life. If the physiological basis for each kind of emotional feeling were known we might have a more satisfactory classification, comparable in definiteness to the classification of sensations. I shall not try to present the best possible classification, but will present the essentials of four different classifications, each arranged by an eminent psychologist. The first to be given is that of Professor Baldwin. A description of the different classes may be found in his *Elements of Psychology,* pp. 241-298.

Baldwin's Classification.—

The Common Emotions

A. Interest.
B. Reality Feeling and Unreality Feeling.
C. Belief.
D. Doubt.

The Special Emotions

A. Of Activity.
  I. Of Adjustment. Distraction or confusion, abstraction or clearness, contraction or effort, expansion or ease.
  II. Of Function.
    1. Of Exaltation. Freshness, triumph, eagerness, alertness, hope, courage, aspiration, elation.
    2. Of Depression. Hesitation, indecision, anxiety, timidity, melancholy, irritation, fear.
B. Of Content.
  I. Presentative.
    1. Self-Emotions.
      a. Emotions of Pride.
      b. Emotions of Humility.
    2. Objective Emotions.
      a. Expressive.

A. Of Attraction.[1]
Admiration, veneration, awe, attachment, affection, confidence, patience, security, etc.

B. Of Repulsion.[1]
Unattractiveness, objectionableness, disdain, distrust, distaste, scorn, rebellion, hatred, abhorrence, contempt, disgust, etc.

b. Sympathetic. Congratulation, fellow-suffering, pity, jealousy, sensitiveness, and many others.

II. Relational.

1. Logical. Feelings of reasonableness and unreasonableness, anticipation, distance, co-existence, quality, identity, fitness, objective power, etc.
2. Conceptional.
   a. For System in Mental Construction.
   b. Ethical Feelings. Moral sympathy, moral obligation, remorse, etc.
   c. Aesthetic Feelings.
      (a) Lower or sensuous.
      (b) Higher or representative.

Wundt's Classification.—It is possible also to classify emotions according to the prominence in them of pleasantness or unpleasantness, of excitement or depression (sthenic and asthenic emotions), and of tension or relief. We can, that is, rate an emotion according to these three scales and group together those which have similar ratings. By excitement and depression are meant the qualities that stimulate or lower general bodily activities. By tension is meant the quality that stimulates the voluntary muscles to over-action and constrained action, by relief the quality that predisposes to free and relaxed

[1] With reference to future and past we have under B2 a A, *hope* and *joy*, and under B2 a B, *dread* and *sorrow*.

action. Glee would be distinguished from joy as being more exciting though not necessarily more pleasant. Both joy and glee would be mediocre with respect to the tension-relief quality. Horror would imply much unpleasantness and tension and some depression. Grief would imply more depression but less tension.

The quality of relief is *per se* pleasant and is ordinarily associated with still more pleasantness. The reverse holds of tension. Both excitement and depression may be accompanied by pleasantness or by unpleasantness. Joy is exciting and pleasant. Anger is exciting, but often unpleasant. Melancholy (in the poet's sense) is depressing but pleasant. Of depressing and painful mental states the number is of course legion.

Royce's Classification.—Another grouping (that of Professor Royce) is according to the pleasantness or unpleasantness and the restlessness or quiescence of the feeling. This latter scale is perhaps a composite of the excitement-depression and tension-relief scales.

Titchener's Classification.—Finally, a still different view is given in the following quotation (for a fuller account see, *An Outline of Psychology,* by E. B. Titchener, pp. 224-234):

"The Forms of Emotion.—Just as there are two kinds or classes of feelings, so there are two of emotion; the pleasurable and the unpleasurable. Within each kind or class there are a large number of special emotive forms, as there are a large number of special 'feelings.' Can we name these forms, and so classify emotions, as we classified sensations and ideas? Or must we be content with the general distinction of the two classes, as we were compelled to be in the case of feeling?.....All emotions are coloured by the organic sensations set up during the adjustment of the physical organism to the situation. If, then, we could find typical groups of organic sensations—lung, heart, bladder sensations—appearing in the various emotions, we could, again, determine the fundamental emotive forms. Our 'physical' would be supplemented by a truly psychological classification.

Although there is no reason to suppose that the problem is insoluble, it has not yet been solved."

Emotions Concerned with the Manner of Thinking.—The feelings which Professor Baldwin describes under the heading, *Relational,* are worthy of special attention. It may be a question whether such feelings of the tendency, direction and attitude of thought should be called emotions, but at all events they exist. We feel in our thinking, not only objects and their relationships and meanings, but also feelings of their comings and goings, of their fitness to our purposes, and of our attitudes toward them. Like the feelings of relationships described in § 11, these feelings of tendency and intellectual attitude are commonly transitive, evanescent, intangible feelings that color rather than compose our mental life. Examine, for instance, the feelings of expectancy, of a mental gap to be filled, and of familiarity.

"Suppose three successive persons say to us: 'Wait!' 'Hark!' 'Look!' Our consciousness is thrown into three quite different attitudes of expectancy, although no definite object is before it in any one of the three cases.

Suppose we try to recall a forgotten name. The state of our consciousness is peculiar. There is a gap therein; but no mere gap. It is a gap that is intensely active. A sort of wraith of the name is in it, beckoning us in a given direction, making us at moments tingle with the sense of our closeness, and then letting us sink back without the longed-for term. If wrong names are proposed to us, this singularly definite gap acts immediately so as to negate them. They do not fit into its mould.

Again, what is the strange difference between an experience tasted for the first time and the same experience recognized as familiar, as having been enjoyed before, though we cannot name it or say where or when? A tune, an odor, a flavor, sometimes carry this inarticulate feeling of their familiarity so deep into our consciousness that we are fairly shaken by its mysterious emotional power."[1]

The Aesthetic Emotions.—The so-called aesthetic emotions also deserve additional comment. The common classification of them is merely into feelings of the beautiful, of the sublime and of the comic. It is obvious that without great straining these three types of feeling fail to include the feelings one has say in seeing an ordinary play or reading an ordinary story. The plays, Sherlock Holmes and Uncle Tom's Cabin, are hardly beautiful, are certainly not sublime and are comic only in spots if at all. Robinson Crusoe is certainly neither beautiful nor sublime nor comic. A more exact division of the aesthetic emotions is evidently needed.

The two main classes of feelings which are meant by the term *aesthetic emotions,* as it is used in critical studies of art and literature and music, are *Sensory Pleasures* and certain *Pseudo-Emotions.* These sensory pleasures are distinguished from the non-aesthetic, first in that they are unselfish, not proprietary, do not imply the possession of, or exclusion of others from, the object causing the pleasure but only its presence; and second, in that they arise from intrinsic qualities of the object, not from its derived values. The pleasures of taste are thus not called aesthetic because one cannot eat his cake and leave it for others to eat too.

[1] W. James, *Principles of Psychology,* vol. I, pp. 250-252.

The pleasure one has in seeing a coin because of its form and chasing is called aesthetic, while the pleasure in its money value is not.

The pseudo-emotions[1] are distinguished from their real correspondents in that they do not arouse the same bodily reactions and impulses and are free from excessive pain or pleasure. Thus the sorrow felt for the suffering hero in the story is unlike real sorrow (1) in that one does not rush around wringing his hands and seeking to offer help nor feel like doing so, and (2) in that, whereas real sorrow is very uncomfortable, the pseudo-sorrow of the reader of the story is more or less enjoyable. In place of both the violent pangs and delights of real jealousy and affection, the reader of a novel has only a rather mild excitement, which is commonly pleasant regardless of the quality of the corresponding real emotion.

§ 16. *The Attributes of Emotions*

Their Bodily Expression.—Omitting from consideration the feelings of tendency and the aesthetic feelings, one finds that emotions as a class are characterized by emphatic bodily expression; *e.g.*, fear expresses itself far more than does a feeling of seventeen. It is usually not difficult to tell whether a person is frightened, happy, angry or eager by his facial expression and bodily movements, whereas it is impossible to tell whether he is thinking of seventeen or of seventy, of a cat or of a mat. Other mental states do, of course, influence the bodily organs, the facial muscles especially, but not to such an extent as do the emotions. Doing arithmetic does raise

[1] It is conceivable, and has, I believe, been by some literary critics suggested, that these pseudo-emotions occupy the same position with respect to real emotions that mental images do with respect to percepts. They are on the whole rather a mystery.

the pulse, but it cannot make the heart go pit-a-pat as fear does. Attention leads to a frown, but not to the tremendous wrinkles of the man in a rage.

Their Impulsive Power.—Emotions, especially the coarser ones, cause not only these expressive movements, but also further movements of effect. They tend to arouse some emphatic acts, running, jumping, seizing, biting or the like. Our ideas and judgments more often guide and restrain, while the emotions more often arouse, action. The more intellectual feelings also, in so far as they do arouse action, lead to the more orderly and restrained movements of face, eyes and throat; while the emotional states impel to more gross and violent movements.

Their Early Development.—The emotions are older in the individual and in the race than images, feelings of meaning and relationships, or judgments. They come along with vague sensations, as early steps in the growth of the infant's mind. During the first year anger, joy, impatience and other emotions are evident. They appear in animals below man in the scale of development. Birds and mammals that give few signs of the possession of images and almost certainly lack feelings of meaning, relationships or judgments, manifest many of the coarser emotions of the human mind. It is when we are absorbed in emotional feelings that we act more or less as the lower animals do. In general the progress of development involves a weakening of the coarser animal-like emotions and their transformation into sentiments by the mixture of ideas with them.

The Infrequency of Reproduced Emotions.—Emotions are less often and less easily imaged than are percepts. One can easily remember that he did feel angry; but he then has not a real image of the anger feeling, but only a judgment that at such and such a time he was angry. Occasionally individuals do have, or at least report that they have, a feeling of anger as not present comparable to the image of a sight or a sound. But such cases are surely rare and may really be cases where the individual by recalling certain circumstances gets a real but lesser emotion of anger, not a true image of it. It may be, as was hinted in the note on page 81, that the revival of an emotion in imagination takes the form of the pseudo or aesthetic emotions.

Exercises

1. Name one or two emotions characterized by much excitement.
2. Name one or two emotions characterized by much depression.
3. Name one or two emotions characterized by much tension.
4. Name one or two emotions characterized by much relief.
5. Name one or two emotions characterized by much restlessness.
6. Name one or two emotions characterized by much definite bodily feeling.
7. Name one or two emotions characterized by little definite bodily feeling.
8. Name one or two emotions characterized by much outward expression.
9. Name one or two emotions characterized by little outward expression.
10. Name one or two emotions which are common to man and the lower animals.
11. Name one or two emotions which are primarily individual, that is concern chiefly oneself.
12. Name one or two emotions which are primarily social, that is concern chiefly others.
13. What is the bodily expression of rage?
14. " " " " " " fear?
15. " " " " " " grief?
16. " " " " " " joy?

17. (a) What part of speech almost invariably expresses an emotional state?

(b) What parts of speech almost never do?

18. What kind of sentence almost always expresses an emotion?

19. Which can animals express to us most clearly, their sensations or their emotions? Why?

References

A. James, *Briefer Course,* XXIV.
Stout, *Manual,* 276-311, 562-580.
Titchener, *Outline,* §§ 31-34, 56-60, 86-91.
Angell, *Psychology,* XVIII.

B. Ebbinghaus, *Grundzüge,* §§ 51-54.
James, *Principles,* XXV.
Wundt, *Physiologische Psychologie,* XVI.

CHAPTER VI

Mental States Concerned in the Direction of Conduct: Feelings of Willing

§ 17. *Definitions and Descriptions*

In General.—Books on psychology commonly announce three divisions of mental life, cognition, emotion and volition, or, in the older phraseology, the intellect, the feelings and the will, but give nine-tenths or more of their space to cognition and the emotions. In so far as psychology attempts merely to describe states of consciousness, this subordination is not unfair. For, although the will in a broad sense deserves as much study as the intellect, states of volitional consciousness, that is to say, feelings of willing, do not require lengthy explanation. For their description this one section will suffice. The will, in the broad sense of the entire basis of human action, will receive due attention in Part III.

The important mental states concerned primarily in the direction of conduct are usually stated to be feelings of *impulse, wishing* or *desire, deliberation, motives, decision* and *choice, will, effort, consent,* and of the so-called *'fiat.'* It is, of course, true that mental states of all sorts may appear in intimate connection with the life of action. But it will be best to follow the custom that singles out for treatment under one head the mental states named.

Impulses.—One is tempted to desire a special name

for the class of feelings which in the round-about phrases of common thought and speech are called 'an impulse to sneeze,' 'an impulse to laugh,' 'an impulse to run,' and the like. Many mental states are so intimately connected with acts that the only names for them are names of the acts to which they lead. *E.g.*, the feelings that lead us to yawn and to cough appear almost never save as impulses to these acts; are not felt by themselves; do not reappear as images; and play but a slight part in the development of the fabric of ideas and judgments as a whole. Yet strictly speaking these two feelings are sensations, are feelings of bodily condition comparable to the sensations of tickling, heat, cold, pain, and the like. And in a strict classification there need be no separate heading for impulses. The feelings that are commonly called impulses are those sensations and emotions which are vague, obscure and little emphasized in the mind in comparison with the acts to which they lead.

It is further true that any mental state whatever may be an impulse,—may take on the aspect of impeller to an act. Feelings of relationships and feelings of meaning do so but infrequently and slightly; images and memories do so somewhat more; percepts, sensations and emotions do so most of all. Those among the last that do so pre-eminently are commonly called impulses.

Although we must abandon the notion of impulses as a group of feelings distinct from all others, we might have a right to speak of an impulse-quality which could add itself to any feeling, but was itself a new kind of mental stuff. But the psychologists of to-day deny that one has that right. By the impulsive quality of a mental state is meant, they say, not any peculiar aspect of it as felt, but only its quality of being connected directly with an act. The description of this impulse quality comes then under the description of the connections between mental states and bodily acts.

Desires and Wishes.—Desire and wishing are emotions, and have been so classified in the previous chapter. When we feel, 'I wish I had that picture,' the feeling includes the thought of the object and an emotional attitude toward it. The particular sort of emotion is, it is true, somewhat more frequently and emphatically connected with conduct than are emotions of other sorts, but the difference is only one of degree. The 'I wish' represents a state of mind not in general character different from 'I hate' or 'I pity' or 'I fear.' It represents a special activity of the mind no more and no less than do they.

Deliberation.—The word deliberation is used in ordinary speech to mean any state of mind in which some topic is considered attentively. It then means little more than a state of attention. In the more restricted use of the word to describe a state of will, psychologists mean by it the consideration of a topic calling for mental choice or bodily action. In such cases the state of mind is likely to include different and more or less opposed motives. We think over the alternatives, have ideas favoring this, that or the other, and swing suspended between them. The presence of percepts, images and feelings of meaning plus an emotion of doubt or uncertainty describes deliberation from the inside. From the outside, it is a state of hesitation before action.

Decision and Choice.—The termination of this hesitation, suspension or conflict of ideas is sometimes marked by a feeling of decision or choice. We must not confuse here the fact of decision with the feeling of decision. The *fact* of decision or choice, which means simply that one motive has conquered,—that one idea or act has prevailed in the mind,—may have much or little or no *feeling* of choice accompanying it. Thus, in writing the last sentence, I thought first of writing 'little or nothing' and then of writing 'little or no.' The latter was chosen, but there was no *feeling* of choice or decision,—no consciousness of anything but the two phrases and the grammatical superiority of the second. On the other hand we often have an intense feeling of acceptance of the one course and of rejection of the other, a feeling of 'yes to this, and no to that.' Such feelings are akin to, if not identical with, the feelings of belief and disbelief and of attraction and repulsion and belong properly among the emotions.

The Fiat.—The term, the *fiat* of will, is applied to a feeling which may perhaps be analyzed ont in some cases from the feeling of acceptance, a feeling of 'Go ahead,' 'Let the act occur,' 'Let the consequences of my decision become real.'

Willing.—The verb *to will* is used as a general term to express the fact of decision in favor of or consent to any course of action which has been the topic of thought. The word is used especially of cases where the decision is accompanied by a feeling of effort, where we decide against natural tendencies. We do not say that we willed to breathe because no decision was involved. We do not say that we willed to eat our breakfast this morning because the action was not the topic of thought. We do not often say that we willed to stay in bed this morning because, though the issue may have been the topic of thought and a decision may have been involved, the action accepted was easy and natural, We do say, 'I got up this morning by sheer will,' because thought, decision and effort were markedly present. In all this there is no description of any special feeling of willing or volition, but only of a general experience involving certain feelings and tendencies to action. The feelings present when one wills to do or think something are in fact those already described.

The Will.—The phrase *the will* is used most often to mean the source of all purposive action. In this sense it equals the general fact of connections between mental states and acts. Thus we say, 'To educate the will is more important than to educate the intellect.' It is used at times to mean the power to inhibit attractive in favor of less attractive ideas and acts. Thus we say, 'It required will to do that.' It is used at times by psychologists as a class name for all those feelings which are closely associated with acts. Thus we say that mental states comprise states of thought, states of feeling and states of will, or are divided among cognition, emotion and volition or will.

The terms *effort* and *motive* have been used without description. The feeling of effort needs no description, for anyone who has ever attended to an uninteresting piece of mental or bodily work, or chosen the disagreeable, repulsive duty, or willed to do and done the painful task, has had direct experience of the feeling. The term motive is used for any sensation, percept, image, feeling of meaning, judgment or emotion which shares in swaying one's decisions. In so far as it influences our willing, any idea is called a motive.

On the whole the feelings concerned in the life of conduct are in the main, perhaps entirely, made up of intellectual and emotional stuff. Action itself *is not* thought nor emotion, but it is *felt in and guided by* thought and emotion. The special psychology of the will is chiefly not a descriptive account of the feelings connected with conduct, but an account of capacities for and habits of action and of the connections between thoughts and acts. This will be found in Part III.

Exercises

Notice your feelings as you follow the directions given in this paragraph. Follow them without question. a. Choose a certain number between 100 and 200. b. Will to turn to that page (*i. e.*, the page of the chosen number) or not to do so. c. It is left to you whether you will take the trouble to write to the author[1] of this book a description of how you feel (a) when you decide to go to church rather than to stay at home, and (b) when you will to continue studying, though bored and sleepy. The information is seriously and earnestly requested by him. Decide whether you promise to do so or not.

1. Did you or did you not in choosing the number have any feeling of decision or of indecision?

2. In case you willed to turn to that page, what was your feeling of willing to do so? (*i. e.*, describe the feeling).

3. In case you willed not to turn to the page, what was your feeling of willing not to do so? (*i. e.*, describe the feeling).

4. In case you decided to promise to write to the author, describe your feeling of deciding to.

5. In case you decided not to do so, describe your feeling of deciding not to.

As before, follow the directions, noticing your feelings.

d. Take a pencil and write your name.

e. Make up your mind to buy ten cents worth of stamps to-morrow.

6. Did you, before taking the pencil and writing your name, (I) feel nothing but the words read; or did you (II) have an image of the movements to be made; or did you (III) have a visual image of the name as written?

If you had any other feelings as components of the 'willing,' what were they?

7. Did you, in resolving to buy the stamps, (I) feel nothing but acquiescence to the words read; or did you (II) feel 'All right,' or 'Yes,' or 'I will'; or did you (III) feel also an image of yourself handling out money; or did you (IV) feel also yourself going to the purchasing place, taking out money and handing it over to the clerk; or did you (V) feel, in place of III and IV or

[1] The author will indeed be very glad if some of the students of this book are willing to send him descriptions of their feelings of willing. He has already many such records.

in addition to III and IV, an image of the stamps as in your possession?

8. In view of your answers to questions 1-7, would you agree with the theory that an anticipatory image of the movement to be made or of the result of the movement was a necessary feature of willing? Would you, for instance, say that the following account was true of all people?

"My volition to sign a letter is either an image of my hand moving the pen or an image of my signature already written, and my volition to purchase something is an image of myself in the act of handing out money or an image of my completed purchase —golf stick or Barbedienne bronze." M. W. Calkins, *Introduction to Psychology*, p. 299.

References

A. Titchener, *Outline*, §§ 36-37.
Angell, *Psychology*, XVII.

B. Ebbinghaus, *Grundzüge*, § 55.
Wundt, *Physiologische Psychologie*, XVII.

CHAPTER VII

General Characteristics of Mental States

§ 18. *Qualities Common to all Mental States*

Complexity.—The fact that one's mental state at any moment is usually a complex mixture has already been emphasized. As the reader sees this page, he feels the temperature of the room and the well or ill-being of his body, thinks of the meanings of the words in this paragraph, has flitting images of this or that called up by them and is mildly interested or bored or satisfied or disgusted with it all. Even if we take but a momentary bit of his mental state it may contain many of these different elements. Although, to study the body of thought and feeling of a human life, we dissect it out into this, that and the other specially named kinds of mental facts, we must not forget that in reality a mental life is a series of confused mixtures of thought-stuff, a rich blending of various elements, and that often all the names so far given to denote different sorts of mental facts would be needed to describe the mental state of a man for a single minute. Mental life is not like a series of solos, now sensations, now memories, now decisions; but is like the performance of an orchestra in which many sounds fuse into a total. One instrument may predominate for a while, but only very rarely is it active alone.

Personal Feeling.—Again, although for convenience we study images, concepts and all mental facts as if one image of a tiger was like another of the same tiger, one feeling of eight like another feeling of eight, it must be borne in mind that what we call the same thought or feeling in two men is, after all, never the same. John in imagining a tiger feels it as a tiger not present and so does James, but John feels the feeling as *his,* as belonging with the rest of his inner life, as a part of his stream of thought. James could feel the feeling just as John does only by being John. If a hundred scholars are asked to add four and four, the hundred thoughts of eight are never absolutely alike. Each eight is felt with a fringe or halo of personal possession,—as someone's own object of thought,—with a tag which says, 'This is *my* thought or *my* emotion.' To quote Professor James:

"In this room. . . .there are a multitude of thoughts, yours and mine, some of which cohere mutually, and some not. . . . . .

"They are as little each-for-itself and reciprocally independent as they are all-belonging-together. They are neither: no one of them is separate, but each belongs with certain others and with none beside. My thought belongs with my other thoughts, and your thought with your other thoughts. Whether anywhere in the room there be a mere thought, which is nobody's thought, we have no means of ascertaining, for we have no experience of its like. The only states of consciousness that we naturally deal with are found in personal consciousnesses, minds, selves, concrete particular I's and you's."[1]

This personal element varies in amount in the same individual at different times and amongst individuals. When one is playing with interest a game of skill or absorbed in the effort of landing a fish or stalking a deer the personal element is almost absent. It is far less in young children than in developed minds. There is

[1] W. James, *Principles of Psychology,* vol. I, p. 225 f.

less and less evidence of it as we progress down through the animal kingdom to the lower forms.

Social Implications.—That in human beings generally thoughts and feelings are always some one's own should not be taken to mean that one man's thought is incomparable with and uninfluenced by those of other men. The likeness of the hundred feelings of eight is far greater than the difference. The isolation of my stream of thought from others is only such that I cannot be them, not such that I cannot be incessantly and to the utmost extent influenced by them. 'Individual' would be a very unfit adjective to apply to human thoughts and feelings if it were to mean more than 'felt always by someone as his own.' So far they are individual, but they are also in an important sense social.

If we leave out any solitary from birth whom chance or miracle may have preserved, the thoughts and feelings of any man at any time are in part the result of the thoughts and feelings of others. What we feel, how we think, what we enjoy, depend on the existence and action upon us of the thoughts and feelings of other people. When the attempt is made to explain the actual mental life of men so as to show how they come to be what they are, the social aspect of mental facts,—the importance of the fact that anyone's thoughts and feelings are members of a great community of mental states,—is abundantly evident.

Mental States are Parts of a Continuum.—Any mental state is felt as a part of a total stream of feeling, as in a context, as with what has been and is to be. The first thought of the morning is thus bound to the life of yesterday, feels at home with the memories of the past and already half-acquainted with the life of the future.

Are, More or Less, Focal.—Thoughts and feelings

may be ranked in a scale according to the degree to which they are absorbing, exclusive of others, impressive characters in one's mental history. A thought may be so prominent, so in the focus that for the time being it practically *is* the mental life, or it may be just a shadowy, almost unnoticed hoverer in the background of the mind.

Within any mental state also some parts are more emphatic, more in relief, gain greater possession of us, count more, are attended to more than others. Psychologists make use of the fitting epithets *focal* and *marginal* to express this unevenness in the emphasis of different parts of a mental state. In the reader's mind the thought, 'more emphatic, more in relief, gain greater possession of us, count more,' should just now have been the chief, focal, absorbing part of his total state of mind; the sight of the rest of the page and the feeling of the book in his fingers less so; while the feelings or noises about him, of the time of day or of the floor beneath his feet should be out in the margin of thought, a shadowy background, half lost in the darkness of the border-land between consciousness and unconsciousness.

If a mental state is pictured as an elevation above the level of unconsciousness, it must be pictured not as a cube or cylinder but as a mountain, the peak representing the focal or attended to part of the thought, the slopes the marginal part merging gradually into the flat plain of unconsciousness. If we picture it as an illuminated area in darkness, the light should be unequally diffused, strong at one point but melting off gradually into darkness.

This general characteristic of thinking by which one thought prevails over others or some one element of a total thought outweighs all the rest is of tremendous practical importance. Not what we think but what is focal in our thoughts, becomes thus the matter of consequence in mental life. This focalizing of thought, commonly referred to by the word attention, will be the subject of a special section.

Other Qualities.—(1) Thoughts and feelings may also usually be ranked in a scale of intensity. Some have an extreme amount of a striking, incisive, piercing quality; others are mild, flat, weak, lukewarm. (2) It may perhaps be possible to rank all thoughts and feelings on a scale of desirability and intolerability ranging from the feeling one most shrinks from to the feeling one most welcomes. This scale, desirability to intolerability, is not identical with pleasure to pain. Certain pleasures may be intolerable and certain pains welcomed. (3) No one could build a pile of feelings over which one could not jump, or fill a bucket with ideas; they do not occupy space. (4) They do take time; as quick as thought is no truer than as slow as thought.

So much for the general inner qualities of mental facts. They have also two general outside relationships. They are intimately connected with conditions of the brain which precede, accompany and, in the common sense use of the word, cause them. They are also intimately connected with acts of the body which, in the common sense use of the word, are caused by them.

These two general facts that all mental life is connected with the activity of the brain and always expresses itself in bodily action will be discussed in Parts II. and III.

Exercises

Experiment 8. The Duration of Mental Processes.—With the proper apparatus for making delicate measurements of time and for eliminating the influence of other processes than those which we wish to measure, the time required to notice a difference, or to call up an image, the time that an idea or an emotion lasts, and the like, may be measured.

Even with the crudest means the differences in duration of the following processes may be at least roughly measured:—

To feel a stimulus and make a movement in response to it.

To feel a stimulus, distinguish it from other possible ones, and make a movement in response to it.

To feel a stimulus, feel its meaning, call up an idea in response to it and make a movement in response to this idea.

Arrange for ten or more individuals to act as subjects: have ready a stop watch measuring fifths of a second. Let the subjects be seated in a circle, the observer among them.

A. Say, "We are to measure roughly the time it takes to hear a sound and make a sound in response. I shall say, 'Be' and as soon as I say it, the person at my right will reply by making the same sound 'Be'; as soon as he says it, the person on his right will make the same sound, and so on around the circle as fast as we can until I say 'Stop'. Be careful not to say 'Be' until you hear the person just at your left say it." Give one round of practice. Then say 'Attention', and then say 'Be', starting the watch simultaneously. After the word has been passed around the circle three times, that is, when you hear 'Be' the fourth time, stop the watch instead of saying 'Be' a fourth time, and then say 'Stop'. If there are ten people the total time taken divided by 30 will be the average time taken to hear the sound and to make the sound and for the sound wave to pass from one person's mouth to the next person's ear.

B. Say, "We will now measure the time it takes to hear a sound, distinguish it from others and make a sound in response to it. I shall start counting, say, with two; as soon as I say two, the person on my right will say three; as soon as he says three, the person on his right will say four; as soon as he says four, the person on his right will say one, and so on, one calling for two as its reply, two for three, three for four, and four for one. Continue until I say stop." Give one round of practice. Then say 'Attention', and say 'Two' or 'Three', starting the watch simultaneously. Stop after three rounds of the circle as before. Compute the average time as before. It will be well to have some one outside the circle watch for erroneous responses.

C. Say, "We will now measure the time it takes to hear a word, distinguish it, think what thing it means, think of some thing connected with this and respond. I, the first person, will say the name of something; the person at my right will reply by saying the first word called to his mind by the word I say, the person at his right will reply by saying the first word called to his mind by the word the second person said, and so on. Be careful to listen only for the word spoken by the person at your left and to reply with the word it calls up." Give one or two rounds of practice and then after the 'Attention' say 'House' and start the watch simultaneously. Stop after three rounds of the circle as before. Compute the average time as before.

Experiments A, B, and C may be repeated as many times as is convenient.

References

A. James, *Briefer Course,* XI.
Stout, *Manual,* 71-76.
Titchener, *Outline,* §§ 92-98.
B. James, *Principles,* IX.

§ 19. *Attention*

The Fact of Attention and the Feelings of Attention.—The words and phrases 'attend,' 'attentive,' 'absorbed in,' 'give one's mind to,' and their synonyms, like most common words, have many shades of meaning. They refer at times to what I shall call the fact of attention and at other times to what I shall call the feelings of attention. In the first case they mean (1) the fact that some part of one's state of mind is focal, prominent, prepotent over the rest or (2) that some one possible idea is noticed and felt to the exclusion of others. Thus (1) 'He attended chiefly to the color of the rose he was observing,' and (2) 'He attended to the rose, not noticing what was said or how awkward he appeared.' In the second case they mean (3) the feeling of effort which so often accompanies the prevalence of one part over other parts of a feeling or of one feeling over others if the natural impulse is to attend otherwise, or (4) the feeling of interest which so often accompanies such prevalence if it is in accord with natural impulse or (5) the feeling of activity,—of oneself being a helper in making the part or idea prevail. Thus (3) 'He resolutely attended,' 'The power of attention;' (4) 'He was absorbed in play,' 'It attracted my attention,' 'I could not help feeling attentive;' (5) 'I was thinking hard. Every sense in me was on the *qui vive*.'

Separate words should be used for each of these five meanings if we are to be clear, at least in all cases where the context does not show in which sense the word attention is used. Let us use *Focalness of Mental States* for the fact that each mental state is not throughout equally prominent, but that parts are in greater relief than others, and *Selectedness of Mental States* for the fact that out of many feelings felt by no means all are noticed, dwelt upon, allowed to play leading parts. For the three chief feelings that accompany such focal and selective thinking, let us use the terms: *The Feeling of Effort or Strain, the Feeling of Interest or Attraction,* and *the Feeling of Activity or of Mental Life.*

(1) and (2) are the most alike. They represent the results of the same mental law acting (A) within one mental state and (B) among a number of mental states. Together they represent the *fact* of attention as opposed to the *feelings going with it.* When in this or later chapters the word attention is used alone it will mean this fact of attention.

Cases of attention may be classified:—

(A) According to the kind of feeling accompanying them, into voluntary and involuntary.

(B) According to the reason why the chief thought

or feeling is chief, into native and acquired, and also into immediate and derived.

(C) According to the nature of the chief or prepotent or 'attended to' object, into intellectual and sensorial.

Voluntary and Involuntary Attention.—In certain cases the special emphasis on some part of our total thought or possible thought is accompanied by a feeling of effort or strain, a feeling of holding ourselves down to that part and resisting other temptations. If in the mind of a schoolboy, in spite of tired eyes and a strong desire to be outdoors, the xs and ys of the algebra book before him hold the field against the shouts and laughter of playmates outside and impulses to look at the clock, to leave the examples till next day and the like, the case is presumably one of voluntary attention. The boy probably has a feeling of effort. Such cases of attention with a feeling of effort are called *Voluntary Attention.* The name is perhaps ill chosen; for in a sense these are just the cases where we do *not* attend willingly. The word voluntary is used by psychologists to show that in these cases of attention with a feeling of effort there is a willful ruling out of other tempting ideas and an adherence to the point attended to.

In other cases an idea is in the focus,—is selected,—without being accompanied by any feeling of effort. On the contrary the object seems to attract us, is more tempting than any others, and is usually accompanied by a feeling of attraction. Such cases are called cases of *Involuntary Attention.* To say that a thing attracts us is simply another way of saying that it wins a place over other thoughts without any feeling of effort on our part. When the percepts of an exciting game hold the field in the school-boy's mind and keep down and out the thoughts of xs and ys, nouns and verbs, sitting still and looking at books, it is presumably a case of involuntary attention. He probably feels little effort in the process.

The feeling of effort of voluntary attention is a feeling arising not so much from thinking of the one thing to which we feel we must attend as from checking or, in technical terms, *inhibiting* the tendencies to think of other things. The real task of the boy in school who with effort keeps the example uppermost in his mind is to keep down and out ideas of how long it is before school ends, of the base ball match in the afternoon, of how thirsty he is, and the like. Thinking and action are of themselves desirable, natural and involuntary; the effort is *not* to think the more attractive thought, *not* to do the more enjoyable acts. It is what we do *not* do that is hard. The fatigue which is in school the so common result of work demanding attention is due largely to the strain of suppressing attractive tendencies. In proportion as the work itself is attractive and absorbing, fatigue diminishes.

Although voluntary and involuntary attention are diametrically opposite, the same object may at one time arouse voluntary attention and at another involuntary. The boy who in the primary school attended to the letters in a book only with effort comes later to read without effort. The song which a few months ago won our involuntary attention has by repetition lost its attractiveness and we listen to it only with a decided feeling of strain. What interests one ceases to do so if no profit or pleasure to him results. What originally implied a feeling of effort becomes freed from it in porportion as profit or pleasure to the mind concerned results.

Other names for *Voluntary* and *Involuntary Attention* are *Forced* and *Free.*

Native and Acquired Attention.—Certain thoughts

and feelings take a prominent place in the stream of thought apart from any experience on our part of their pleasurableness or utility. The inborn constitution of human beings is such that in young children a clear, bright light wins a place in the focus of the mind over filmy shadows,—that the sight of a puppy running about excludes the feelings of the clouds or trees. The fact of attention in such cases is called *Native* or *Inborn Attention* because it is caused by inborn qualities.

In the majority of cases of attention in adult life, however, the tendency for the uppermost idea to be uppermost has been caused by our experiences of the different ideas concerned and of their consequences. The black and white of printed pages gains attention because of the pleasures that have come from reading, the utility of the information gained and the like. The dollars and cents, clothes and furniture, concerts and plays, the spoken and written words, which figure so largely among the prominent, focal, attended to ideas of civilized human beings do not owe their prominence to the inborn constitution of man, but to the circumstances of his life and training.

Cases of native attention are always involuntary. There is no feeling of effort in doing what one's inborn make-up leads him to do. Cases of acquired attention may be voluntary or involuntary.

Immediate and Derived Attention.—A less useful division is into *Immediate* and *Derived Attention,* immediate attention meaning those cases where the prominence of the object is due to some intrinsic quality of its own, and derived attention meaning those cases where it is due to some thing not in the object but indirectly associated with it. The attitudes of a baby and of an adult toward a twenty dollar gold-piece are cases in point. The first is immediate attention due to the glitter of the form itself;

the second is largely derived attention, due to the ideas connected with twenty dollars. The reason why this division into immediate or intrinsic and derived or extrinsic is less useful is that it is in many cases extremely hard to decide which occurs. For example, does the miser attend to the gold for itself or for its indirect properties? Certainly the attention was originally derived, but certainly it feels to him now immediate.

Sensorial and Intellectual Attention.—Cases where the object that is prominent is a thing of sense are called cases of *Sensorial Attention.* Cases where it is an image, meaning, concept, or the like, are called cases of *Intellectual Attention.* Thus 'His mind was absorbed by the face before him,' gives an instance of the former, and 'His thoughts were firmly fixed on the idea of self sacrifice,' gives an instance of the latter. Many other divisions could be made, according to the nature of the object of attention, into attention to thoughts and attention to acts, attention to feelings of external things and attention to feelings of the body, etc.

In common use the word attention refers to physical facts as well as to mental facts. 'I attended to the lectures' means in common speech not only 'Percepts of the words spoken were predominant among my feelings and excluded other feelings,' but also, 'My eyes were directed toward the lecturer and followed his movements. They focussed upon him, not upon something in front of or behind him. My ears were held tense as in listening.' The connection between the mental fact attention, which this chapter has dealt with, and its physical or bodily expression, to which the word attention so often refers, will be discussed later in its proper place.

Attributes of Attention.—Much has been written about the extent to which one idea in the focus of thought may shut out others. Even the most intense stimuli may fail to influence one who is thus absorbed. Stock illustrations are the soldier who, absorbed in the excitement of the battle, fights on unconscious of severe wounds, the child absorbed in his story book who fails to reply to the loudest call, and the preacher who, although so afflicted with weakness as to have to be carried to his pulpit, yet in the course of his discourse rose from the chair in which he had been seated and soon was speaking with full voice and vigorous gestures. Though such extreme cases of the victory of a possessing idea are rare, the same thing occurs to a less degree with everyone in every day's work. We can and do 'put things out of our mind' by attending to something else.

Whether it ever happens that all parts of a state of mind are equally focal, equally attended to, is a doubtful question. At times, for instance when he lies idly dozing in a hammock, a person seems to feel one thing as much and no more than another, to be equally open to all parts of an impression, to care no more for one element of a thought than for another. But in such cases attention may not be really dispersed equally over the field, but may have run from one thing to another very rapidly. Each element may have been attended to in its turn somewhat exclusively. The question is not of much importance, since such cases are certainly rare in mental life. As an almost, if not quite, universal rule mental life is focalized.

What common usage calls inattention is then very, very rarely real inattention, attention to nothing, but only attention to something else. We call him inattentive who does not attend to what we wish or expect him to. The reason is to be sought not in the non-focal quality of his mental life, but in the fact that it is focussed on something else. The inattentive boy of the school is commonly extremely attentive to the bent pin he is preparing for his neighbor's sleep or to the dreams of out-of-school life which fill his mind.

Analysis.—Closely allied to the fact of focalness of thinking is the fact of analysis,[1] the fact of breaking up a total fact into its elements, parts or aspects. It is only as a result of such a process of breaking up total facts into their qualities that the elements of color, size, shape, weight, pressure and the like are felt in place of a 'big, blooming, buzzing, confusion.' It is only as a result of such a process that many feelings of meanings and of intellectual relationships arise at all. In the fact of focalness of thinking lies the possibility of feeling one part or element of a fact and neglecting the rest. As now the color, now the size and now the shape, of, say, a plate is made focal in the infant's mind, he is able with aid from a law to be described in Chapter XIV to think of the color of the plate, the size of the plate and the shape of the plate each by itself, and to think of the total fact, the plate, as possessing or constituted by these elements.

Exercises

1. Classify each of the following cases of attention as voluntary or involuntary, as native or acquired and as intellectual or sensorial:—
   a. The baby's fixed glance at the bright light.
   b. The miser's absorption in contemplating his hoard of gold.
   c. The poet's attention to the composition of a poem.
   d. The school boy's attention to it in learning it by heart for to-morrow's lesson.

[1] The word discrimination is used sometimes with this same meaning of coming to feel parts of facts, but as it is more often used to mean feeling differences between facts, the word analysis is preferable.

e. The compositor's attention to the copy of it in setting it up in type.
f. The child's attention to the piece of candy held before him.
g. His attention to the organ-grinder's monkey.
h. His attention to the letters in the primer from which he puzzles out the words.
i. The sailor's attention to the sail he can barely discern in the distance.
j. The young girl's attention to the memories of last night's party.

2. Illustrate from your own experience the power of inattention to temporarily banish pain and fatigue.

3. What are some of the things and qualities to which attention is naturally given as a result of inborn constitution regardless of our experience of their effects?

Experiment 9. The Fluctuations of Attention.—Paint a very light gray circle about a half inch in diameter on a square of white cardboard or heavy paper, the color of the circle to be barely distinguishable from white (about 2 drops of black writing ink to a teaspoonful of water will do if painted in a thin coat). Place the square of cardboard far enough away so that the gray circle can just be made out. Look steadily and attentively at it for six or eight minutes. What happens to the gray circle?

Experiment 10. The Relative Time of Focal and Marginal Thinking.—Read passage A not thinking of the words at all attentively: read it, that is, as one skims over an unimportant passage or a perfunctory letter. Keep a record of the number of seconds which elapse. It will be convenient to start when the second hand is at 60. Read passage B attentively, as one would read an interesting book or a notice of importance. Score the time as before. Compare the times.

A.

Passing down the street you come first to a tall, brick building, then to the Presbyterian church, and next to the store of William Gunnison. Above the door hangs the sign, "Antiques Bought and Sold." If you go in you will see tables, chairs, bedsteads, and desks of mahogany, mirrors in gilded frames which Mr. Gunnison will assure you are genuine Chippendale, and an almost endless row of grandfather's clocks. The walls are covered with shelves and racks and hooks on which rest or to which are hung thousands of pieces of crockery of all sizes and shapes imagined and unimagined. Blue, brown and lavender figured plates jostle pewter, china and earthen tea-pots.

B.

Just across the river is situated a prosperous-looking farm-house with a red barn and a little beyond it a grove of pine trees. Near the gate stands a man with sword and pistol. In the house he has stored knives, guns, cutlasses and Indian tomahawks, and ninety Italian stilettos, each of which, he informs visitors, has killed a man. In spite of the murderous nature of Mr. Talbot's mania, he is kind to his horses, cattle and dogs. He simply enjoys collecting weapons as other people enjoy collecting more peaceful objects. He gathers straight, curved and pointed swords and daggers as you might gather pictures, books or oriental rugs.

Experiment 11. The Influence of Attention on Memory.—Write what you remember of both passages, A and B. Compare the results.

Experiment 12. The Aid of Attention in Analysis.—(a). Sound or, better still, have some one sound for you on a piano, a chord made up of the middle C and the note C′, an octave above it. Do you hear the two components or is the sound apparently only one note? If the latter is the case, sound several times the C′ until you have it clearly in mind. Have the chord played again. Do you now hear the C′ as a component? If the chord was felt as a result of two component tones notes from the start, experiment as follows:

(b) Strike the middle C alone. Do you hear any component notes? Strike softly the C′ until you have it clearly in mind and then listen for it as you again strike the middle C. Do you hear the C′ now? The middle C does contain the C′ as one of its overtones and with enough practice and close attention it can be detected.

References

A. James, *Briefer Course*, XIII.
Stout, *Manual*, 611-614.
Titchener, *Outline*, §§ 38-42.
Angell, *Psychology*, IV., 64-82.

B. Ebbinghaus, *Grundzüge*, §§ 56-59.
James, *Principles*, XI.
Wundt, *Physiologische Psychologie*, XVIII. § 1.

§ 20. *A New Classification of Mental States*

The thoughtful and ingenious student may have observed already that human thoughts and feelings may be ranged in a scale according to the directness of their relationships to their 'objects,' that is the things which they stand for.

Feelings Which are What They Stand For.—There are firstly feelings, such as of blue, length, suffocation, sleepiness, terror and rage, which simply *are* what they stand for. These may be called feelings of the first intention. They give us the stuff, the content, the material out of which the mind's world is shaped. They mean or refer to or know nothing unlike or beyond themselves. The suffocation, as a feeling of the first intention, stands for just the suffocation; the blue means just the blue. In adult life one rarely has feelings of the first intention pure and simple. Even the suffocation is felt as, 'I am strangling,' or 'What an intolerable atmosphere,' more frequently than in its bare, intrinsic self. To get adequate illustrations of them one must turn to such feelings as one has when, in close touch with nature, without thought of 'things' or 'self,' he feels impressions directly. Think for instance, of how one feels when half dozing in the summer sunshine or when swimming lazily, or when in the agony of whooping-cough or asthma, or when beside oneself with rage, or when absorbed in the smell of the woods. One is then swallowed up in the sensation, is lost in the feeling, for the time being *is* it. One does not 'think' or have 'ideas' or notice 'things.' One simply feels the warmth, the water and the sky and one's bodily movements, the pain, the rage, the odorous air.

Feelings Which are Like What They Stand For.—There are, secondly, feelings such as percepts and images (and the pseudo-emotions), which have objects, more or less, but always somewhat, like themselves. The feeling of the blue which we call a feeling of 'the sky,' the feeling of a white rectangle which we call a percept of a sheet of paper, the image of the line an inch long—each of these refers to something which it is not exactly but only in part. They may be called feelings of the second intention.

Feelings Which are Unlike What They Stand For.—There are in the third place feelings which may be utterly unlike the facts to which they refer. These feelings of the third intention or symbolic feelings include the feelings of intellectual relationships, of meanings, of judgments and the like. A single illustration will suffice. $(a^2—b^2)=(a+b)\ (a—b)$ is, in so far as it is a feeling merely of the straight and curved lines seen, a feeling of the first intention; in so far as it is a feeling of letters and signs, that is, of certain things or images which the straight and curved lines call to mind, it is a feeling of the second intention: while, in so far as it is a feeling that one means, 'Any *a* squared minus any *b* squared equals the sum of these quantities times their difference,' it is a feeling of the third intention. It is in the third intention that feelings become the rational or strictly human kind of thinking. They can have as objects, things that are not, have not been and cannot be felt in the first or second intention. Millions of lengths that could be so felt only in the course of a lifetime can be felt in the third intention as easily as can a single inch. Differences that are indistinguishable and elements that are indissoluble by direct feeling can be thought. What the eye has not seen nor the ear heard can thus enter the mind of man. Far and near, past and future can be joined in thought. Feelings of the third intention do thus in a sense transcend the limits of space and time and place thought *sub specie* *aeternitatis.* The universe can be and is destroyed and recreated in the mind.

The Attributes of Each of These Classes.—Feelings of the first intention are common to many, if not all, of the members of the animal kingdom. Feelings of the second intention may appear here and there in a few of the higher vertebrates, but in general are lacking in the lower animals. Feelings of the third intention are the exclusive property of man, and fail to appear in the less developed minds of idiots. In the growth of any individual's mind the second class appears only after some months of life, and the third only in proportion as the second becomes established.

Feelings of the first intention are strongly impulsive to bodily acts. As a bone is to a dog's mind literally a 'to seize and gnaw;' as a sunny dust pile is to the chick's intellect literally a 'to scuffle and squat in;' so, to man as well, a feeling of cold is in its first intention a 'to shiver, crouch or get away from.' Whereas feelings of the first intention thus impel to immediate bodily action, those of the second are especially provocative of delayed action, of action only indirectly and after a time. Their direct consequence is more often another idea. The printed *a*, which in the chick arouses only an act, viz., 'to peck,' because the chick feels only the first intention, will in a man arouse the image of the sound of *a* or the ideas of *b*, *c* and *d*. Feelings of the third intention impel to immediate action still more rarely and arouse judgments rather than images. In the long run, however, they influence action more than do the others, for through them we can react once for all to a whole group of objects or to some quality in all the thousands of cases where it is found. In fact the less our thoughts resemble their objects the better they seem to serve us; the less their immediate expression, the greater their eventual influence.

CHAPTER VIII

THE FUNCTIONS OF MENTAL STATES

§ 21. *The Function of Mental Life as a Whole*

Thoughts and Feelings Influence Action.—The function of thoughts and feelings,—*i.e.,* the work they do, the service they perform, their share in the business of life,—is to influence actions. In some wider, freer world than that of this present life, mental states may count of themselves directly. But as things are here, we help or harm our fellow men only by what we do. Only when a man's ideas and emotions issue in effects on his deeds, words, gestures, facial expression or other bodily acts, do they make any difference to anyone else. And in truth, though it would be a long task to explain why, it is only when they influence such acts of body or at least of brain, that they make any permanent difference to him. Unless mental states resulted in acts that altered the physical world or the bodies and minds of men they would be of no service, and would as well not be. In § 27 it will be shown that sooner or later, directly or indirectly, every mental state is expressed or worked off in causing or inhibiting bodily movements or brain changes. That we now see to be their reason for being. We feel the outside world in order that we may react to it. We remember and learn and reason in order that we may *modify* our reactions to it. The great majority or our feelings have as their function *to change our behavior.*

The great majority of our actions are done in response to and under the guidance of mental states. Getting up, dressing, eating breakfast, the work of business or study, the play of games and social life, what we say, where we go,—the entire course of a day's doings minus the merely physiological activities of digestion, circulation and the like,—represent the stimulation to and control of conduct by thought. The history of a man's life of action as a whole is the history of the changes in his natural make-up which have been wrought by his mental life. The steel which always reacts uniformly to the magnet by approach,—the acid and metal which always react by combining to form hydrogen and a salt,—these give no sign that they possess feelings; but in the animal kingdom in proportion as we find the power to change the individual's responses to conditions, to adapt behavior to circumstances, in the same proportion we find evidences of conscious life.

Knowledge Is Not the Sole or Ultimate Purpose of Thought.—It is a common mistake to speak of mental states as a means to knowledge as if that were their final goal. Mental states are not in all cases means to knowledge. Many of our emotions and impulses furnish us only with tendencies to act. For instance, love and envy do not enlighten our minds with respect to their objects but only change our dispositions toward them. When mental states are means to knowledge the knowledge itself is really valuable chiefly as a means to action. It would be of little advantage to have sensations of cold or knowledge of the physiological effects of low temperature if one never was moved thereby to put on a coat or build a fire. The reasoning of the mathematician is well nigh profitless until it is expressed in words or diagrams or some other form of expression so as to influence the world's behavior. We learn so as to do. Thought aims at knowledge, but with the final aim of using the knowledge to guide action.

Adaptation.—Intelligent behavior,—that is, reacting to the situations of life so as to adapt oneself to them,—involves three factors: (1) being sensitive, (2) acting or making movements, and (3) connecting with each of the different situations certain particular movements. We might give these three factors names as follows:—

(1) Sensitiveness or Power of Impression or Reception.

(2) Movement or Power of Expression or Action.

(3) Connection or Power of Association or Elaboration.

We could then say that the function of mental life was to be impressed by the environment and to associate suitable acts with all impressions. The work of education is to make the impressions, acts and connections between them suitable not only in the sense of suiting the actual world but also in the higher sense of suiting the ideal demands which are to transform the imperfect world that is into some better world of the future.

That mental life in general serves to adapt conduct to environment in useful ways does not imply that in each and every case it does so. Feet are useful in general but they sometimes trip us up; the blood is useful in general but it serves at times as the medium for disease. So thought, though useful in general, at times leads men into blunders. That we can swallow food implies that we can also swallow poison, and that we can think wisely implies also that we can make mistakes. Moreover, just as the evolution of the body does not keep pace with the changes in the environment and manifests useless organs such as the vermiform appendix, so also the mind shows useless

8

sensations such as those coming from tickling, useless emotions such as hysterical fear or joy.

I shall not waste the reader's time in the following account of the special functions of different classes of feelings and connections between them by rehearsing under each head the cases of useless functioning. The reader should once for all understand that such exceptions occur. In the text only the more general facts will be presented.

§ 22. *The Functions of Different Groups of Mental States*

The Function of Sensations and Percepts.—The function of sensations and percepts is to serve as signals to warn us of the presence of some thing or quality or condition and so to arouse the appropriate thought or act or emotion. Sensations and percepts may be likened to the signals of an army or the steam-gauge of an engine. They report what occurs within and in the neighborhood of our bodies, that is they report more or less of the environment, and thus are the first step in our adaptations to it. This does not mean that a sensation or percept necessarily resembles or duplicates or mirrors the thing it stands for. The feeling of sweet no more needs to be like sugar than does the position of the indicator on a steam-gauge to be like an explosion. A toothache is no more like a decayed tooth than it is like a green light; a sound is no more like air-vibrations than like ether-vibrations. The function of the sensations is not to give us a picture of the outside world but to lead us to act properly toward it. It is indeed literally true that we in any case sense not so much what is present, as what it is useful for us to feel.

The different sensations give, of course, warnings of

the existence of different qualities or features of physical things or bodily conditions. Sights and sounds are specialized signals of distant objects; pains, of conditions dangerous to life and health; and so on through the list. In general, sensations are warnings that emphasize the presence of qualities and conditions, while percepts are warnings of the presence of things themselves.

The Functions of Images and Memory.—The function of images is to permit us to prepare for future reactions to things not at the time present. They allow us, so to speak, to anticipate the future, to prepare for war in time of peace. By thinking of the frosty Caucasus we can take measures in thought or action against the time when we shall actually confront it. It is by virtue of images that man thinks before and after and so modifies his behavior apart from the stress of immediate contact with things. He can thus spend days in preparation for a situation which in actual presence would allow of hardly a minute's thought. Instead of having to wait for the convenience of nature, he can suit nature to his thought.

The function of the permanence of mental changes in conscious memory and in unconscious habits of thought and action is, of course, to permit experiences to extend their influence into the future. Man and other animals as well would quickly succumb to the environment if the lessons it taught them in one hour were all lost during the next. It would be useless and indeed meaningless to learn if we learned only immediately to forget.

The Function of Feelings of Relationships.—To explain in detail the service rendered by feelings of relationships would require too intricate an analysis of their influence on human conduct. In general they enable man to adapt his reactions to the world as a related whole. Since things are alike and different, are causes and effects, are before and after, are above and below, awareness of these relations guides our reactions to the things. And since the relations often equal or outweigh the things in practical importance, awareness of relations will often be of as great service as awareness of things.

The Function of Feelings of Meaning.—The function of an individual notion is to provide a constant mental sign for one particular thing, regardless of the variations in its appearances in percepts and images. Thus we can mean or think 'John Smith' no matter whether his face or voice or the sound of his name is perceived or imaged. The provision of a constant mental sign to stand for 'John Smith' anywhere and always implies the provision for similar reaction to 'John Smith' anywhere and always. The individual notion then enables anyone to economize by having one reaction to one thing instead of many reactions to its varied appearances.

The function of a general notion or concept is to provide a constant mental sign for any one of the members of a group. As before, this implies the power to react similarly to any member of the group by reacting to the sign that stands for any one of them. Since seven means any seven and five means any five, any seven and any five make twelve. Since acid means any acid and base means any base we can once for all form habits of knowledge and action respecting the union of any acid and any base. General notions are the short-hand of thought.

The function of an abstract notion or abstraction is to provide a mental sign for and hence means of reaction to some element or aspect or quality or relationship regardless of the particular thing or things in which it appears. Thus we react to intentions regardless of results; to lengths without either breadth or thickness; to times apart from anything happening in them; to shapes regardless of what they are shapes of. In a sense we recreate the world to suit us by analyzing it in thought into elements more manageable and by reacting, not to the total situation with which we are confronted, but to some element in it which offers a vital point of attack.

The Function of Emotions.—Emotions serve to emphasize certain things and conditions and to lead to action in more specific and intense ways than do sensations and percepts. They commonly go with those things and conditions which nature has taught us to emphatically seek or avoid. The teachings of nature in this respect are however of much less value in the conditions of modern civilized life than they would be if man were still leading an animal life in the woods. Jealousy and rage, for instance, could be omitted from human life with little loss.

It is often stated that the emotions furnish the energy for action, while the intellectual states only guide and enlighten; that without the emotions man would never act vigorously. This is false. Men of vigorous action *seem* to be moved by strong emotions because acting vigorously itself tends to produce strong emotions, but really clear insight and prompt decision do as much to favor action as do soul-stirring fervor and intense passion. It would be truer to say that strong emotions represent a partial waste of the energy that should be used in action. The waste is only partial; for the emotion does, as was said in the previous paragraph, emphasize the situation and so intensifies action somewhat.

The Functions of Connecting, Selecting and Analyzing Agencies.—It is perhaps needless to call attention to the function of habits, the associations of ideas, and judgments. They are all names for connections; the first a general name, the second a name for connections amongst ideas only and the third for connections commonly between concepts, abstractions and individual notions, connections that also usually involve a felt relationship. The function of connections as a class was made clear in the first few paragraphs of this chapter. Instincts, though also connections having in general the function of all connections, have as their special function that of providing for the essentials of preservation and of serving as the material out of which the edifice of habits is reared.

Analysis, in the sense of noting parts, does the actual work of breaking the direct concrete experiences of things up into elements, and so of producing the abstractions the function of which we found to be so important. In fact the power to 'see into things,' to 'pick out the essential factor in a situation,' is as important practically as the power to 'put two and two together;' so that analysis is as useful as association.

The function of attention, is, first, to economize time and effort. The selective activity for which attention stands concentrates mental life upon the things, qualities, and conditions of moment to us and allows the rest of the universe to slip by without taking our time. It allows us to proportion the prominence any thing shall have in the mind to the importance it possesses for our welfare. In the second place, attention is one main step toward analysis.

Only this brief statement of the functions of the means of connection, selection and analysis is given here, because the same topic will be dealt with more fully in Part III.

Exercises

The function or part played by different features of mental life can be concretely imagined by thinking what would be lost from life by the loss of any one of them.

Thus suppose a man to be:—

1. Without any concepts or abstractions.
2. Without any permanence to his ideas.
3. Without any images.
4. Without any established connections amongst his ideas.
5. Without any established connections between ideas and acts.
6. Without any restriction of thought to special features of the situations encountered.
7. Without any sensations.
8. What are some of the difficulties that would be caused if the feelings of things in memory or anticipation were indistinguishable from the feelings of things present to perception?

PART II

THE PHYSIOLOGICAL BASIS OF MENTAL LIFE

CHAPTER IX

The Constitution of the Nervous System

§ 23. *Gross Structure*

Human thought and conduct are intimately connected with the working of the nervous system, by which is meant the brain and spinal cord, the nerves from these to the organs of sense and to the muscles, the nervous tissue in the organs of sense, and the sympathetic system and local ganglia. Injuries to or diseases of the nervous system cause marked changes in thinking and action. Brain tumors may result in disordered thinking; diseases of certain nerves cause inability to move the corresponding muscles; disease of the optic nerve causes blindness. Drugs which affect the nervous system, such as chloroform, alcohol and hashish, produce mental symptoms. The development of the nervous system in child life parallels the growth of bodily control, intellect and character. From a vast amount of such evidence as this it is abundantly shown that the thoughts and feelings and behavior of men are in direct relations with the activities of the nervous system.

The appearance to the naked eye of the human nervous system, as in Figs. 2, 3 and 4, offers little instruction to the student of mental life. The surgeon or physician must know its shape, the names of its parts, and the outlining walls of its ventricles, because he has to operate upon it. Its more detailed inner structure, as shown by the microscope and by modern histological methods, is of chief concern to the student of psychology. It is not the gross appearance but the composition of the nervous system that throws light upon human learning and conduct.

The reader should, however, in order to understand later descriptions, recall from his studies of physiology[1] that the nervous system as a whole is divided into (1) the central nervous system, (2) the nerves passing from it to different parts of the body, (3) the sympathetic system and its isolated ganglia in different parts of the body and (4) the nervous apparatus of the end-organs (eyes, ears, etc.). The central nervous system is further divided into the brain and spinal cord. The brain is further divided into the cerebrum, cerebellum, medulla oblongata and other parts. The cortex of the cerebrum is the gray matter composing its outside layer.

In the descriptions of the figures, the name refers to the source from which the figure was copied. Barker refers to L. F. Barker's '*The Nervous System and Its Constituent Neurones;*' Edinger to L. Edinger's, '*Nervöse Centralorgane,*' 5 Auflage; Kölliker to A Kölliker's, '*Handbuch der Gewebelehre des Menschen,*' Zweiter Band, 6 Auflage; Lenhossék to M. v. Lenhossék's, '*Der Feinere Bau des Nervensystems,*'. 2 Auflage; Starr refers to the reproductions of M. Allen Starr's series of photographs of the brain's finer structure in his '*Atlas of Nerve Cells*'; Van Gehuchten refers to A. Van Gehuchten's '*Anatomie du Système Nerveux de l'Homme.*' Roman numerals refer to the volume, the first arabic numeral to the page, and the second arabic numeral to the number of the figure in the original.

[1] The student who has never studied human anatomy and physiology should read the chapters on the nervous system in some standard text book of human physiology.

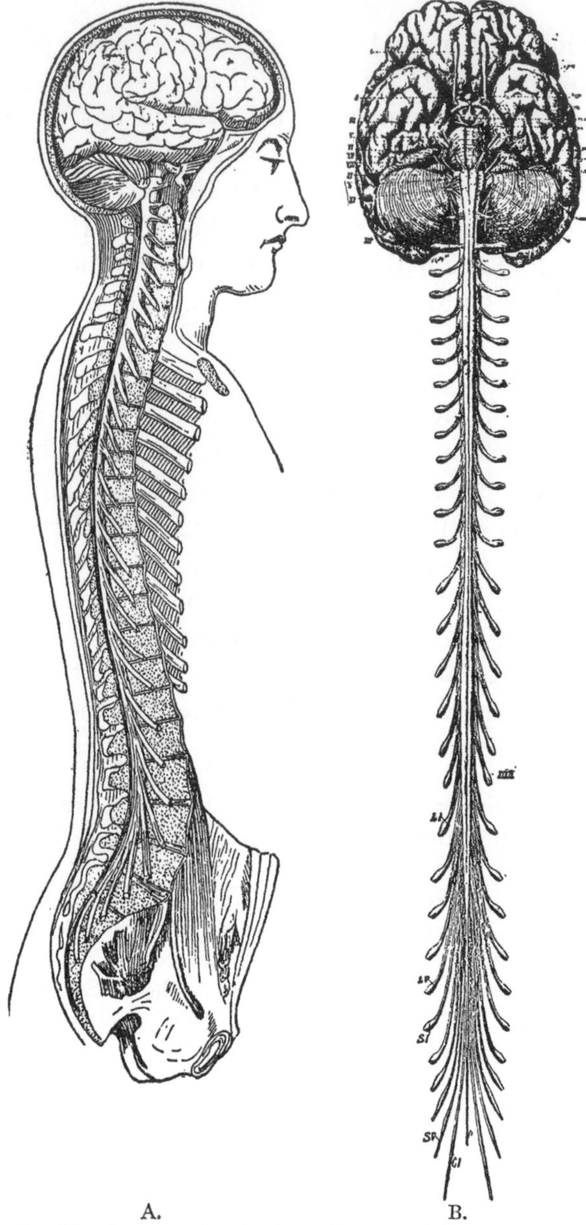

A. B.

FIG. 2. A. The brain and spinal cord, viewed from the side, in their relation to the general structure of the body. One-seventh natural size. B. The brain and spinal cord, viewed from the front. Three-seventeenths natural length After Van Gehuchten, I, 2, 1 and 2.

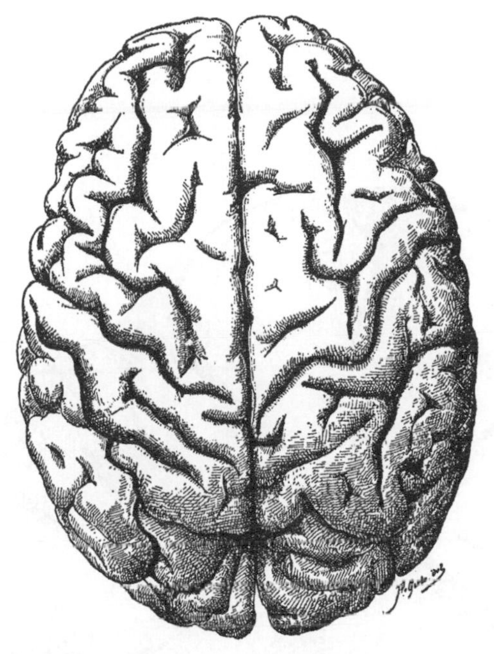

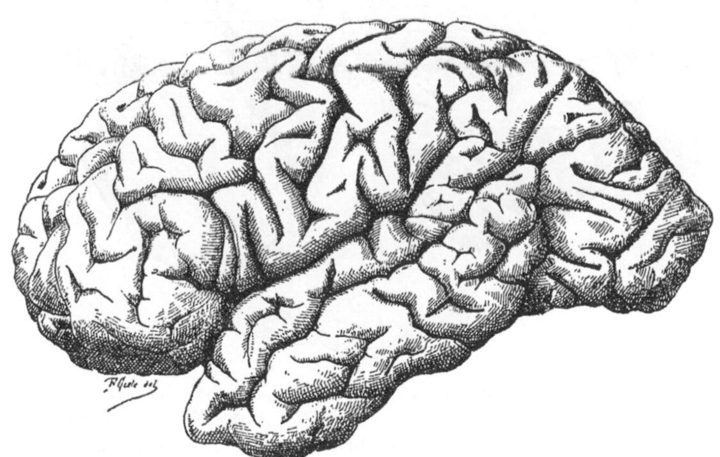

Fig. 3. A (above). The cerebrum, viewed from the top. Two-fifths natural length. After Van Gehuchten, I, 80, 60.

Fig. 3. B (below). The cerebrum, viewed from the left side. Two-fifths natural length. After Van Gehuchten, I, 87, 69.

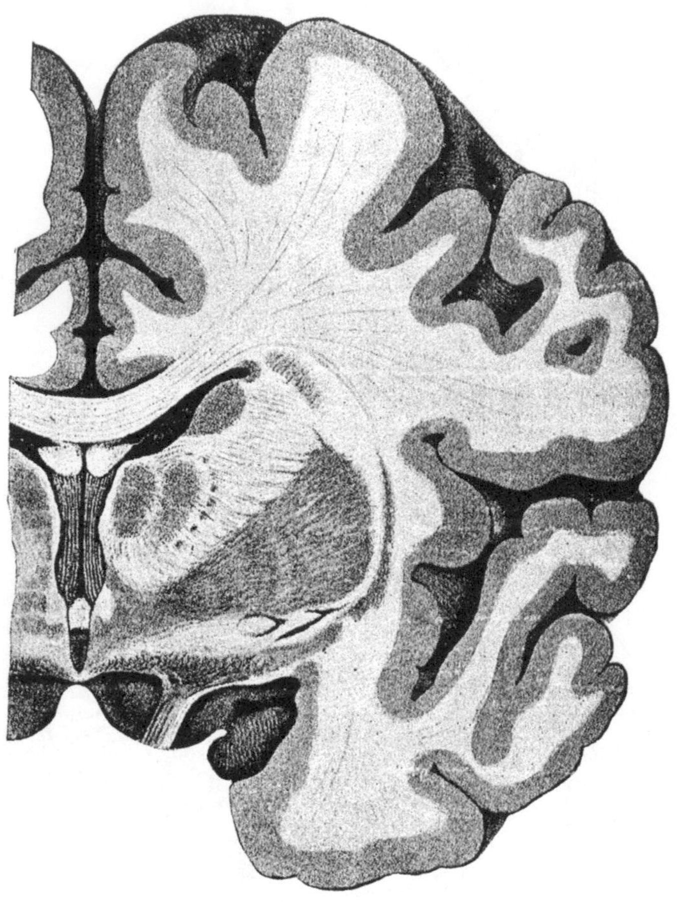

Fig 4. A section through the cerebrum, showing the appearance to the naked eye of the white and gray matter and the relation of the cortex to the inner substance of the cerebrum. After Edinger, 254, 173.

§ 24. *Finer Structure*

The Nervous System Equals the Sum of its Neurones.—The nervous system proper (exclusive, that is, of the blood vessels and lymph which permeate it and the tissues which act as connective and supporting structures) is composed of units of structure called neurones or nerve cells. For instance, the optic nerve is essentially a bundle of very fine thread-like bodies of protoplasm placed side

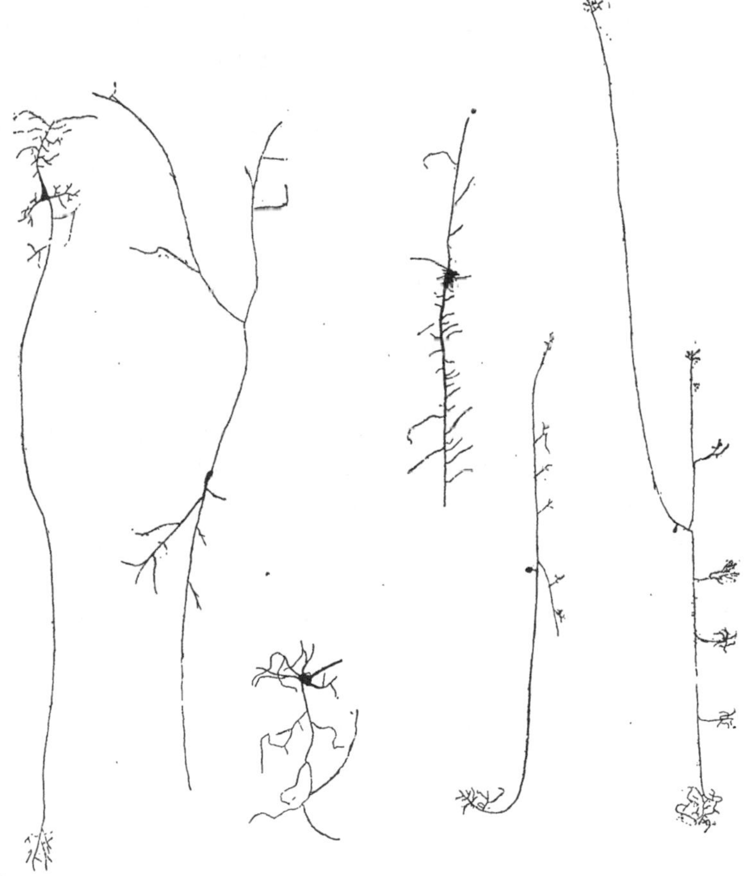

FIG. 5. Rough sketches of six neurones. Thickness is overestimated relatively to length.

by side like the wires running from pole to pole along a telegraph line. Each of these neurones or nerve cells of the optic nerve has one end in the retina of the eye and the other in the brain (in the parts called the geniculate bodies). Again, if we could see exactly the structure of the brain itself, we should find it to consist of millions of similar neurones each resembling a bit of string frayed out at both ends and here and there along its course. So also the nerves going out to the muscles are simply bundles of such neurones, each of which by itself is a thread-like connection between the cells of the spinal cord or brain and some muscle. The nervous system is simply the sum total of all these neurones, which form an almost infinitely complex system of connections between the sense organs and the muscles.

Fig. 5 gives a general idea of the essential features of a neurone, or nerve cell, by giving simplified drawings of several types of neurones.[1] Figs. 6-16 may help to make real the idea that the brain and other components of the nervous system are essentially a vast assemblage of these string-like neurones. Figs. 6-11 are reproductions of drawings made with all possible fidelity to the actual facts; Figs. 12-16 reproduce actual photographs of very thin sections from the central nervous system, so stained as to show its composition. In examining them one must bear in mind that such sections will rarely if ever show the whole of any one neurone, but only cross views of parts of some, lengthwise views of parts of others, here a main string, there a frayed-out end. It is also the case

[1] The student will of course bear in mind that the fraying out is not simply in one plane, that the neurone is not flat. Moreover, in the drawings the thickness of the string and its branches is over-estimated relatively to their length. To get a true idea of these relative proportions in the longest neurones one would need to have a page many yards long or on a page of this size to represent the main string of the neurone as less than a thousandth of an inch thick.

that the method of staining used is such that not all of the neurones are stained. If they were, the whole picture would be a dense-black mass, so closely are the string-like nerve units packed together. The top of Fig. 15 gives some idea of this closeness of interweaving.

If the reader will think of a slice through the brain, such as appears to the naked eye as in Fig. 17 or Fig. 4, as being really of the appearance which a combination of hundreds of such drawings and photographs as Figs. 6-16 would make, he will have a true though crude conception of the general characteristics of the brain's structure. It is absolutely essential that the picture of it as a custard-like mass of gray and white stuff be replaced in the reader's mind by a picture of it as an aggregation of millions of thread-like neurones, each a perfectly definite unit by itself.

The drawings, I repeat, are in no sense unreal or simply general diagrams, but are actual reproductions of the things seen under the microscope. The photographs are of course absolute copies of actual cells as found in sections cut from the brain and stained. It is unfortunate that a picture of an entire neurone cannot be gotten by the camera, and that one sees therefore only a scrap of one neurone here and a scrap of another there. Figures drawn as well as photographs taken give a false idea of the length of the neurone. The longer ones do not appear for the very good reason that at the magnification of say 190 diameters, a drawing of one of the longer neurones would have to be a tenth of a mile long.

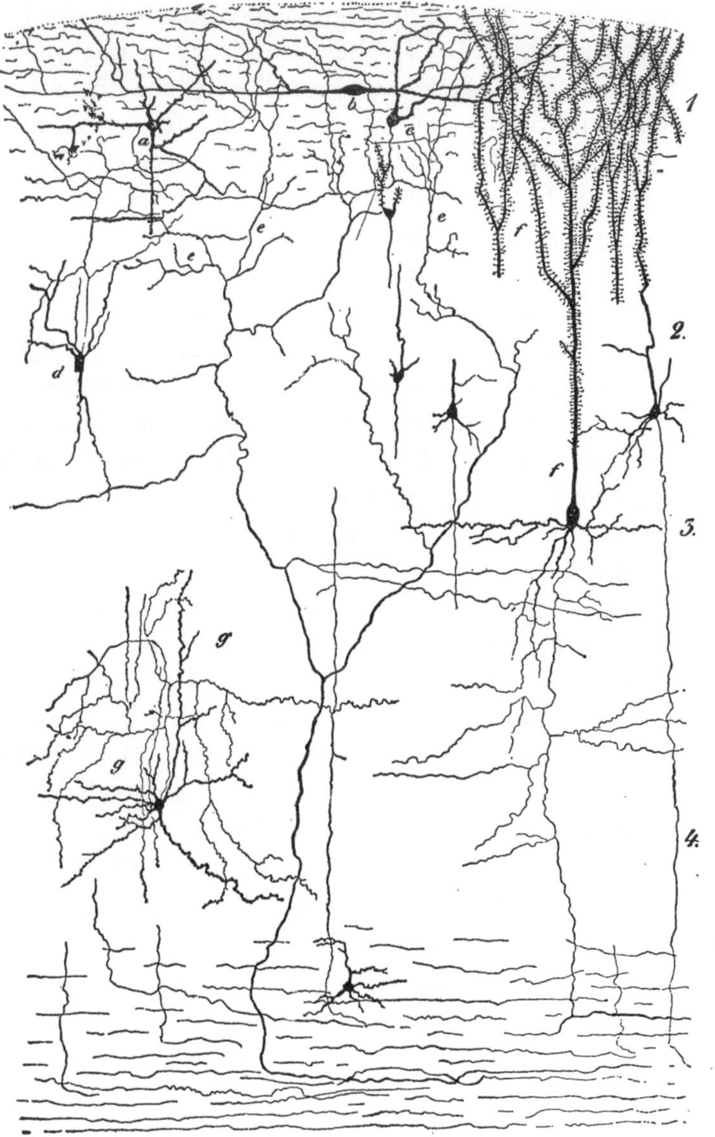

Fig. 6. A sketch showing elements of the structure of the brain cortex in mammals. These are drawn from actual specimens. Greatly magnified. After Edinger, 221, 152.

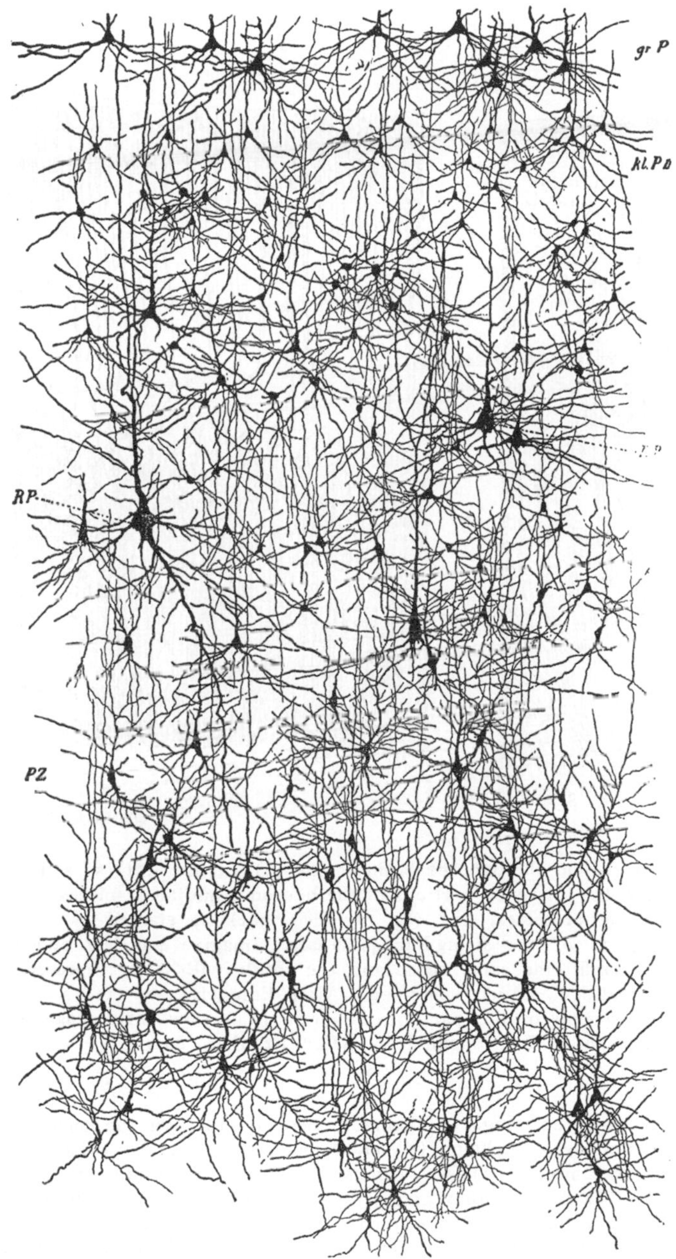

Fig. 7. A section through the brain cortex. Greatly magnified. After Kölliker, 652, 732.

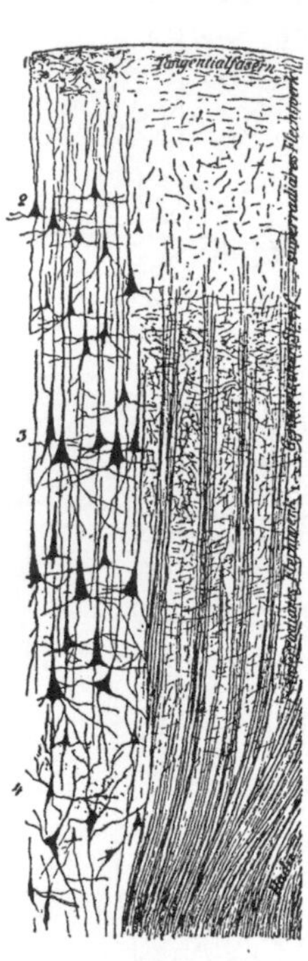

FIG 8.

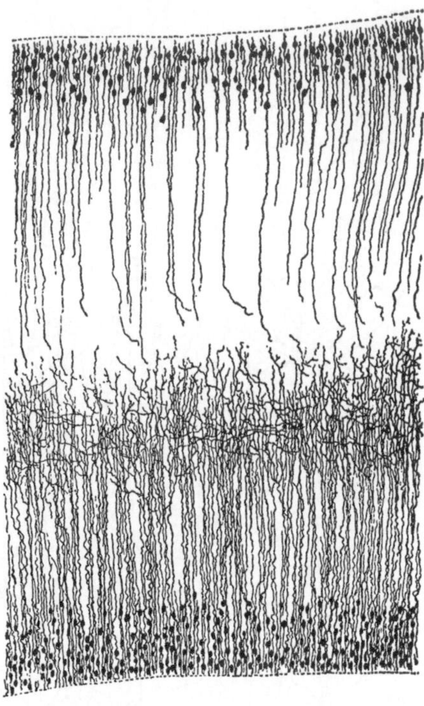

FIG. 9.

FIG. 8. A section through the brain cortex (a) (at the left) so stained as to show the thickened portions of the neurones and short pieces of their string-like processes, and (b) (at the right) so stained as to show only parts of the string-like processes. Imagine the left and right halves to fill the same space and the result will fairly represent the real condition. Much magnified. After Edinger, 220, 151.

FIG. 9. A section of the part of the brain in a very early stage of its development. Much magnified. After Kölliker, 802, 814.

FIG. 10 (above) and Fig. 11 (below). Sections through the medulla oblongata or myelencephalon (the enlargement of the spinal cord where it joins the brain). These sections are from the brain of a young mouse, but the idea they give of the general structure of the brain is perfectly applicable to the human brain. After Van Gehuchten, II, 386, 597 and II, 392, 603. Both figures are due originally to Ramon y Cajal.

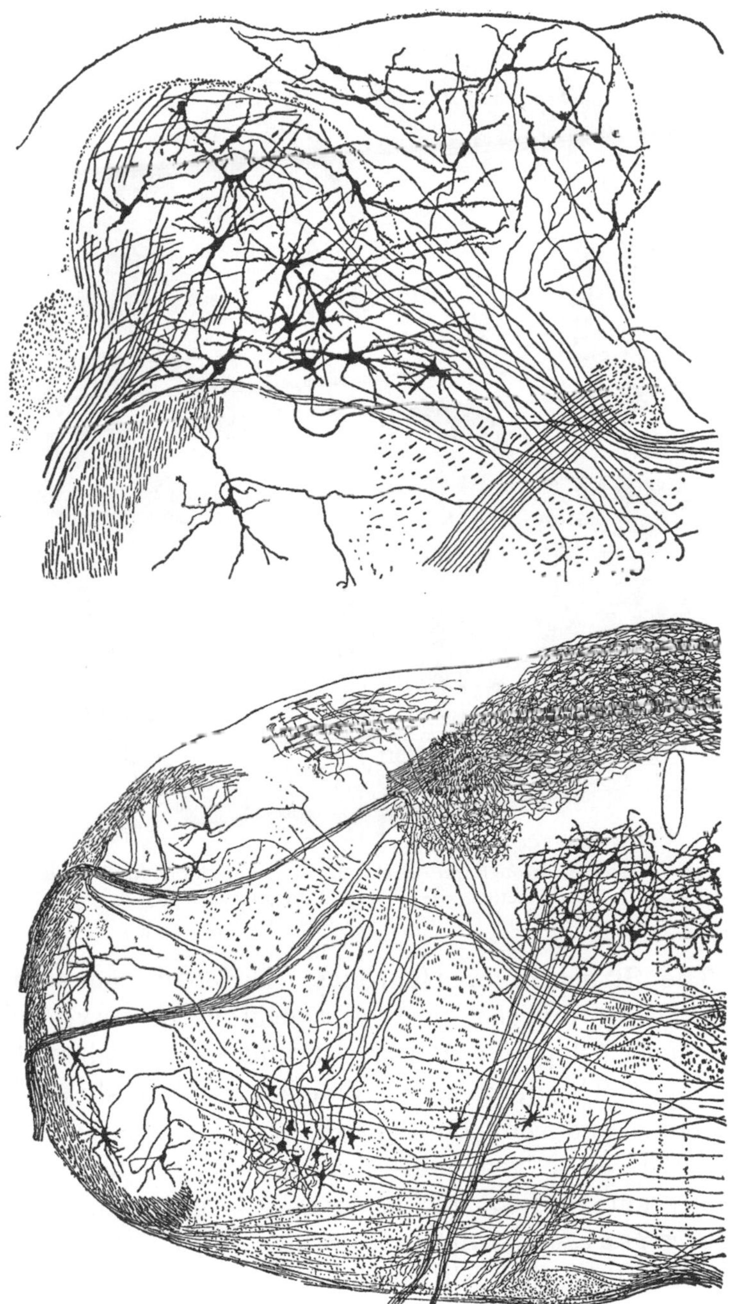

FIGS. 10 AND 11.

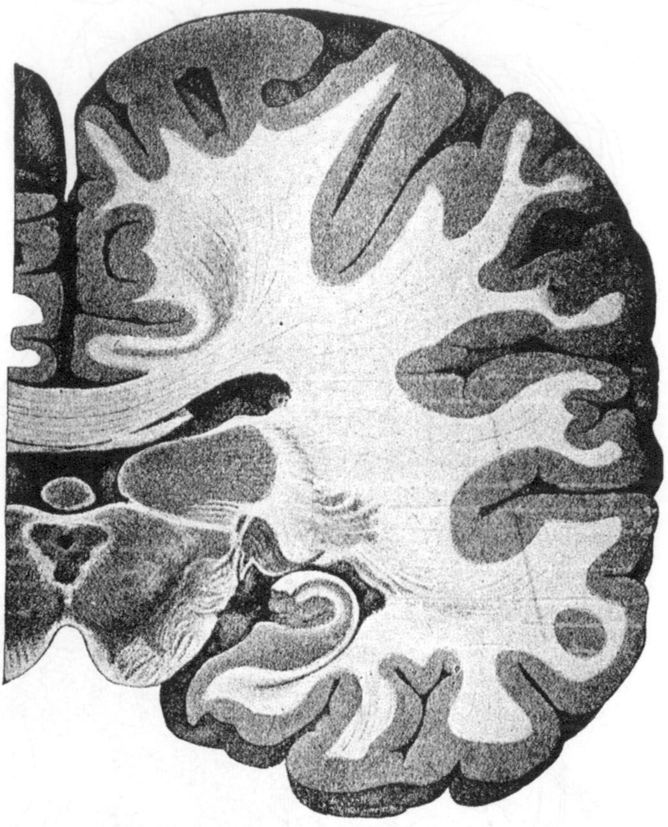

FIG. 17. A section through the cerebrum, as it appears to the naked eye. Nearly actual size. After Edinger, 243, 165.

The Structure of Neurones.—Different names are given to the different parts of a neurone or nerve cell. The thickened part containing the nucleus is called the *cell-body*. The process that diminishes in size slowly in its course and commonly goes a considerable distance from the cell-body and gives off branches rather infrequently until it frays out at its end, is called the *axis-cylinder process* or *neuraxon* or *axone*. The one or more processes that diminish rapidly in size, that commonly

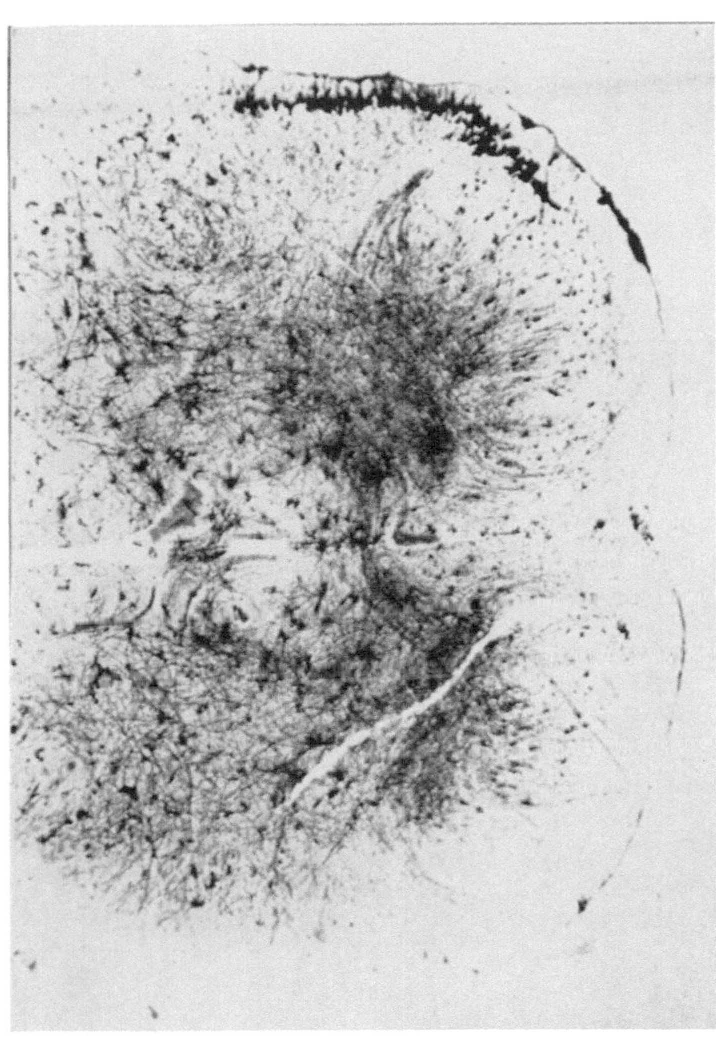

Fig. 12. A photograph of a section of the spinal cord in an early stage of the development of the nervous system. After Starr, 20, Plate 2. ×27 Diameters.

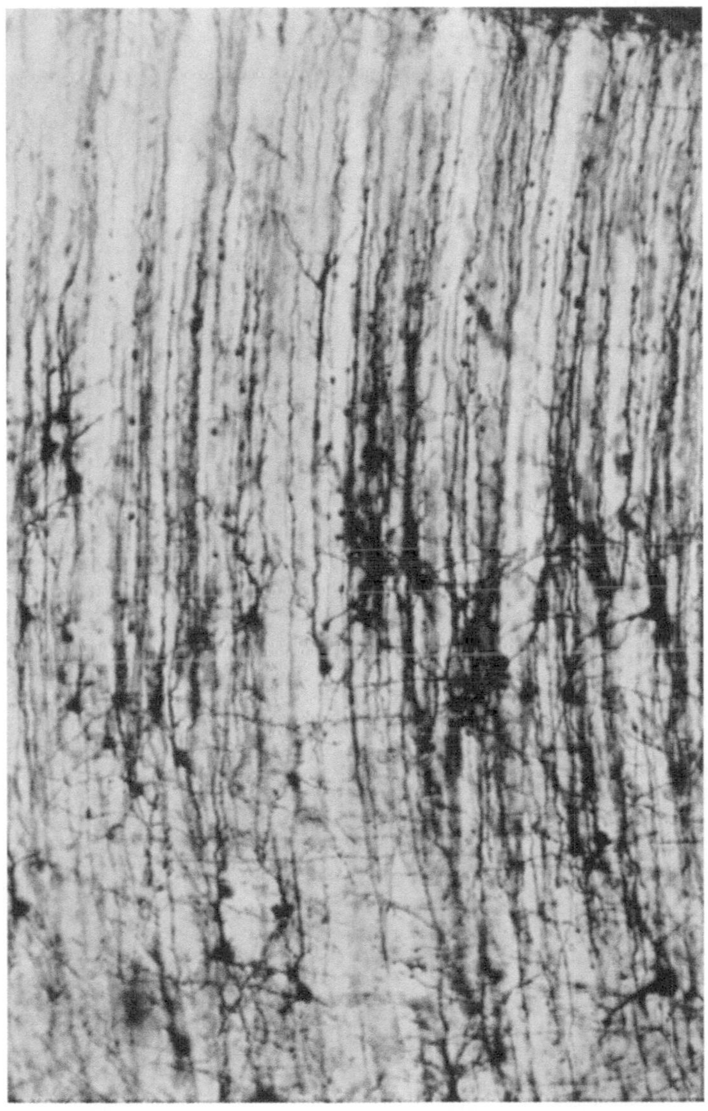

FIG. 13. A photograph of a section through the cortex of the cerebrum, showing segments of very many neurones. After Starr, 68, Plate 41. ×150 Diameters.

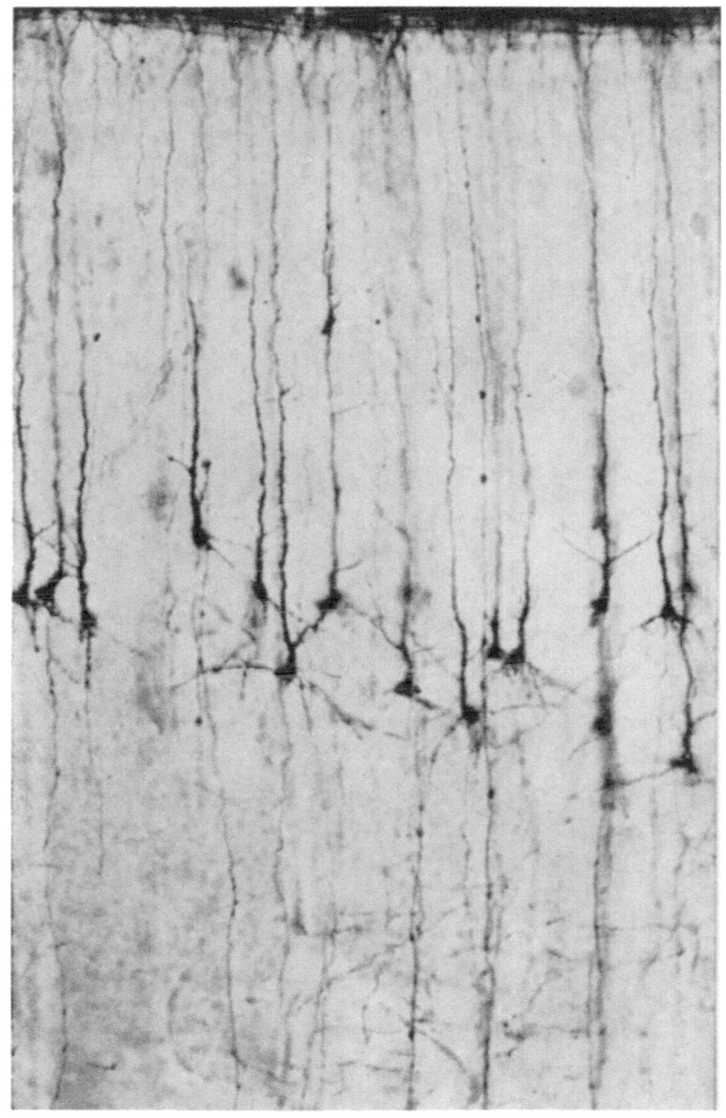

Fig. 14. A photograph of a section through the cortex of the cerebrum in an early stage of development of the nervous system, showing segments of a number of neurones, including the thickened part,—the so-called cell-body of the neurone. After Starr, Plate 42 ×150 Diameters.

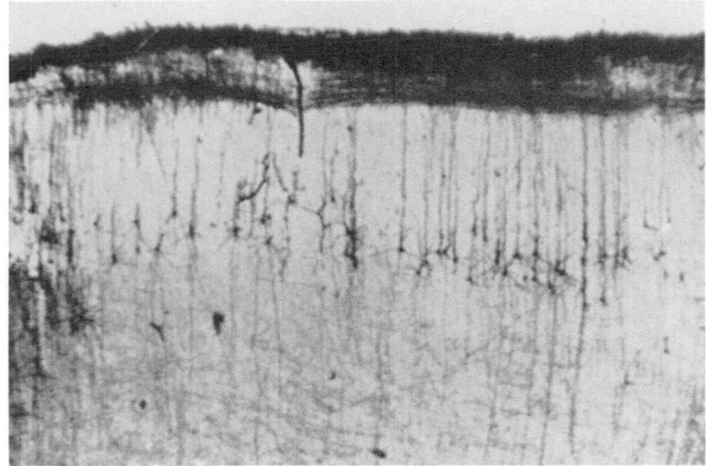

FIG. 15. A photograph of a section through a convolution of the cerebrum in an early stage of development of the nervous system. The black mat at the top of the photograph represents a dense aggregation of the frayed-out ends of many neurones; in the rest of the photograph are seen clearly segments of many separate neurones, with the thickened parts of about thirty in a nearly horizontal line. After Starr, 62, Plate 33. ×20 Diameters.

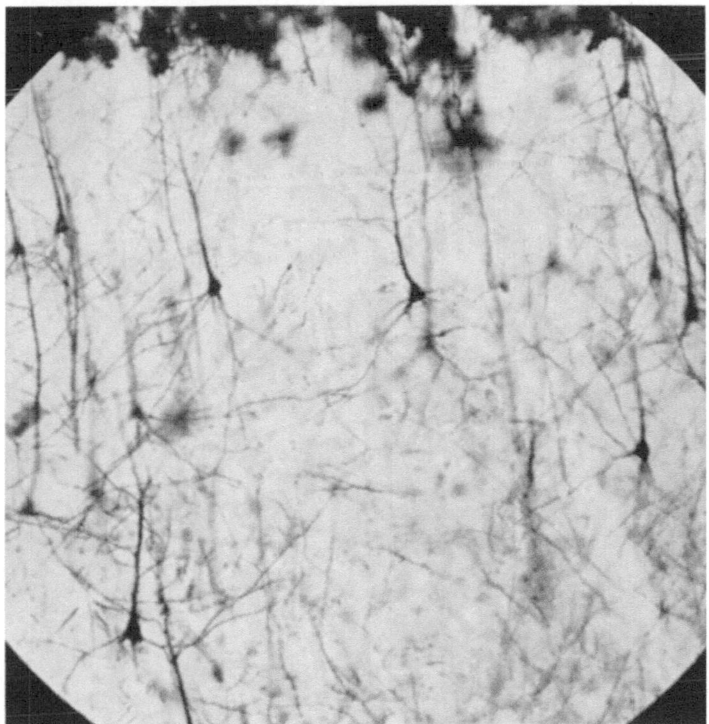

FIG. 16. A photograph of a section through the cortex of the cerebrum, showing short segments of a number of neurones, including in many cases the thickened part,—the so-called cell-body of the neurone. After Starr, 67, Plate 40. ×120 Diameters.

go only a slight distance from the cell-body and branch again and again like a tree are called the *dendritic processes* or *dendrites.*[1] The fine branches given off from

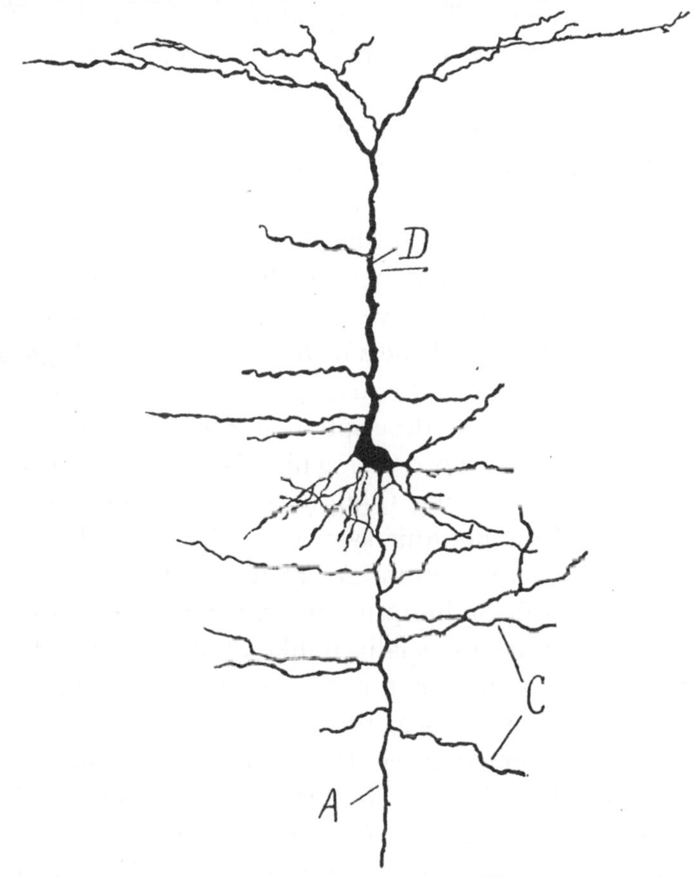

Fig. 18. A neurone from the cerebral cortex. The axis-cylinder process, dendrites and collaterals are marked A, D and C respectively. The neuraxon is shown in the drawing only for a short distance. If its entire length were pictured it would run for yards below the bottom of the page. Very greatly magnified. After Van Gehuchten, I, 201, 145.

the neuraxon are called *collaterals.* The branching out at the end of a process is often called (by Latin words

[1] An absolutely comprehensive and exact distinction between neuraxon and dendrite cannot be made that will agree with the different usages.

meaning the same thing) the *terminal arborization.* (See Fig. 18.) These different parts of the neurone are clearly shown in Figs. 19-23 which represent neurones or parts of neurones. They may also be observed in the actual photographs of neurones reproduced in Figs. 26-29.

The part of a neurone called the axis-cylinder process or neuraxon or axone is throughout a part of its course covered with a surrounding substance or sheath, called the *medullary sheath.* When a part of a neurone is called a fibre, the part of it thus ensheathed is called a medullated fibre. Neuraxons in that part of their course outside the central nervous system have a second sheath outside the medullary sheath, called the *sheath of Schwann.* Figs. 24 and 25 (p. 137), show the arrangement of these sheaths.

It is clear from the description so far given and from the figures that the word *cell* which is used for the unit of structure in any living thing does not describe the unit of structure of the nervous system at all well. The great majority of structural units are at least somewhat like a cell or box or bag or lump in shape, but the 'cells' of the nervous system are especially unlike all other cells of the body and utterly unlike the cell of common language. These may be thousands of times as long as they are wide or thick, are extremely irregular in their shape, and would be far better described by the term, nerve-string or fibre or tangle. The unfitness of the term is one reason why the nerve cell is commonly described as a cell-body plus cell-processes. It has also been the cause of a most misleading habit: namely, the use of the word cell for the cell-body alone and the word fibre or process for the string-like parts of the cell. The student should remember always that the process or fibre is always a part of a neurone or cell, and as important a part as the cell-body. It would be a sad mistake to think of the thickened part

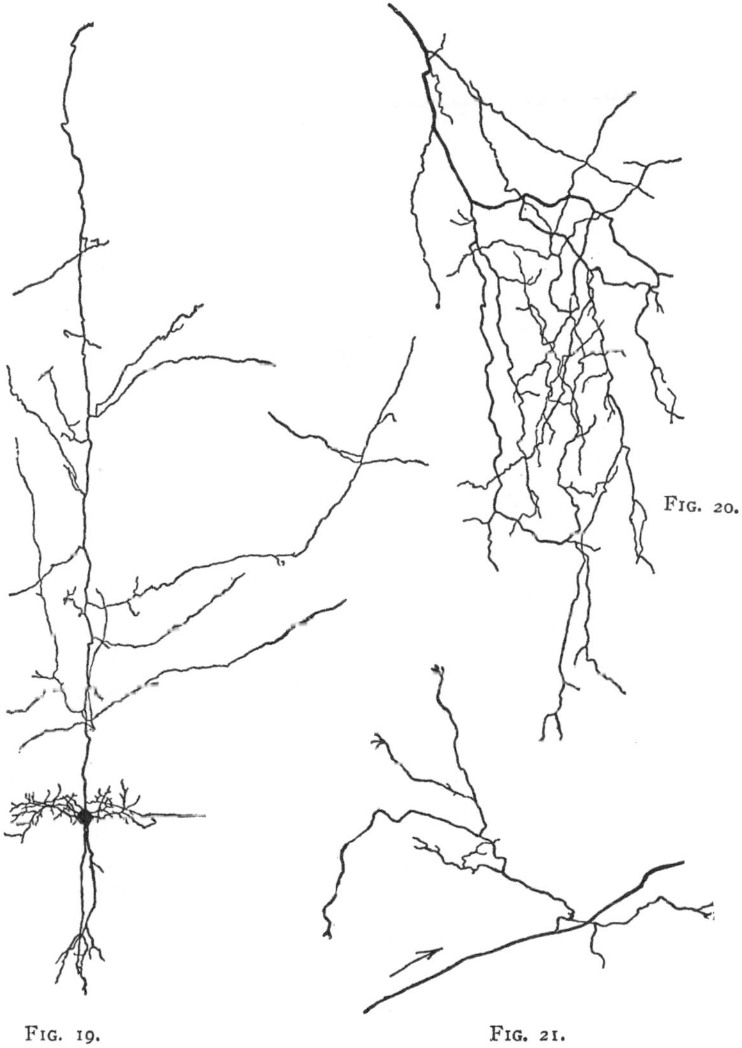

FIG. 19. A neurone from the optic lobe. Very greatly magnified. After Kölliker, 419, 578.

FIG. 20. A segment of a neurone from the optic lobe. Only the frayed end or terminal arborization is shown. Very greatly magnified. After Kölliker, 583, 693.

FIG. 21. A segment of a neurone from the spinal cord, showing a collateral. Very greatly magnified. After v. Lenhossék, 255, 36.

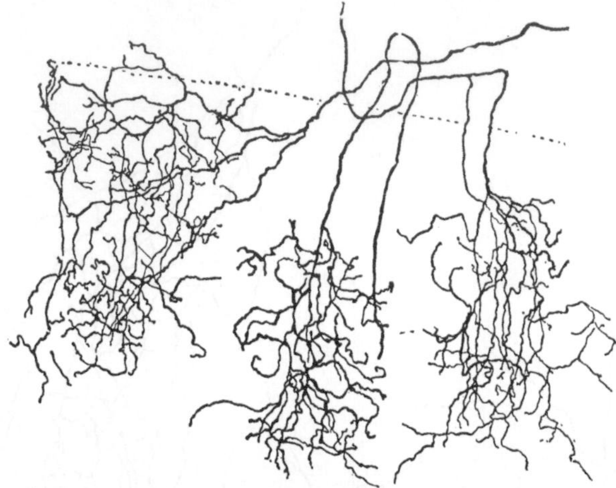

FIG. 22. Segments of three neurones from the optic nerve's termination, showing their frayed ends or terminal arborization. Very greatly magnified. After Kölliker, 416, 575.

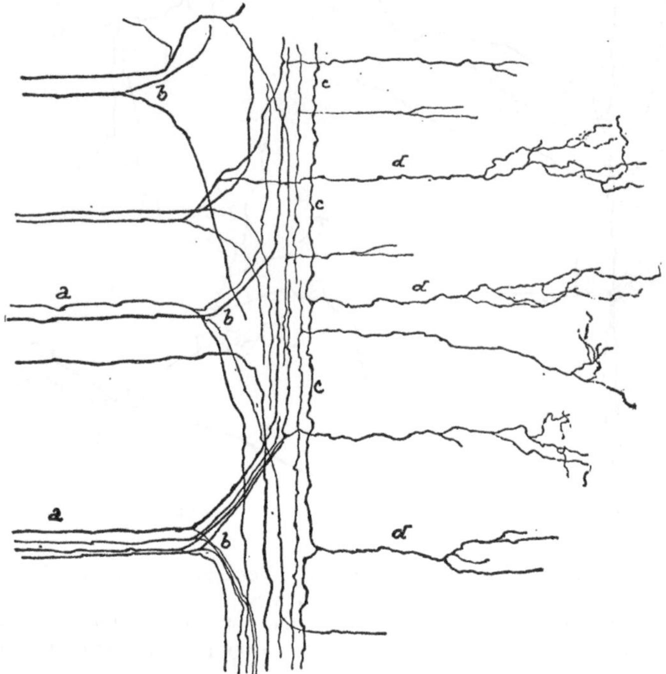

FIG. 23. Segments of neurones from the spinal cord, showing also collaterals (d). Very greatly magnified. After v. Lenhossék, 287, 45.

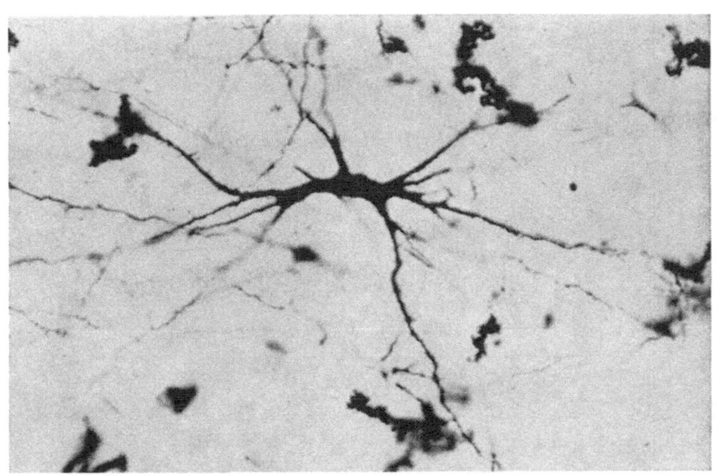

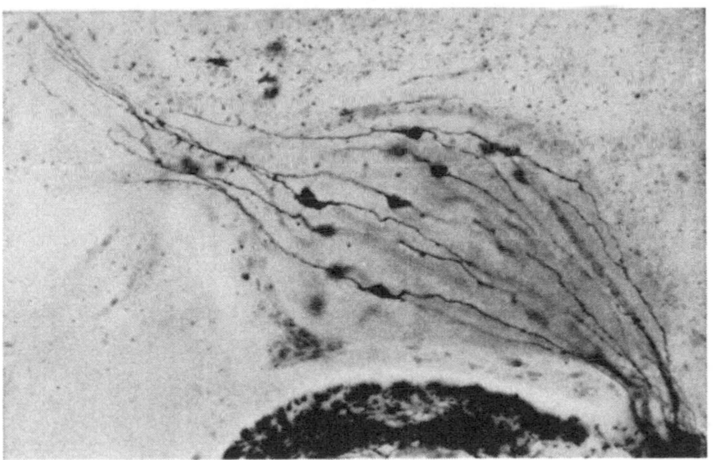

Fig. 26. A photograph of a cell-body of a motor neurone in the spinal cord with numerous dendritic processes and the beginning of the neuraxon. The latter passes from the cell-body at the left hand side and runs almost horizontally to the edge of the figure. After Starr, 21, Plate 3. ×120 Diameters.

Fig. 27. A photograph of segments of several neurones from a spinal ganglion of an embryo chick. The cell-body and the extensions of the neurone from it are very clear in five of the neurones. After Starr, 21, Plate 11. ×120 Diameters.

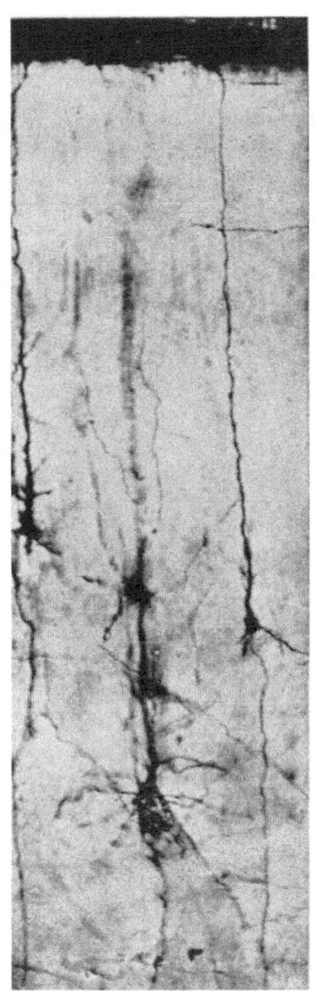

Fig. 28.

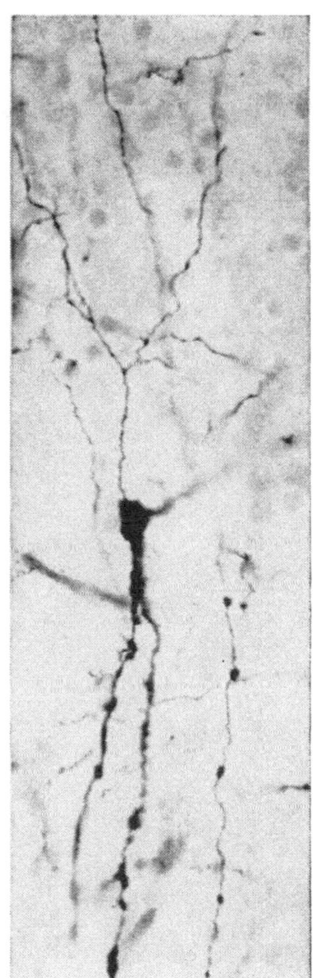

Fig. 29.

Fig. 28. A photograph showing at the right a segment of a neurone including the cell-body, the neuraxon running downward and a long dendritic process running upward to form, by branching, a part of the black mat at the top of the figure. After Starr, Plate 44. ×120 Diameters.

Fig. 29. A photograph of a neurone of the third layer of the cerebral cortex, showing the cell-body, dendritic processes and the neuraxon; the latter runs upward, and divides into two branches which later divide again. After Starr, Plate 46. ×330 Diameters.

where the nucleus lies as the essential, and of the processes or thinner parts as minor features.

The thickened part is not the main thing even in bulk. The process or fibre part is almost always larger, in some cases nearly if not quite two hundred times as large.

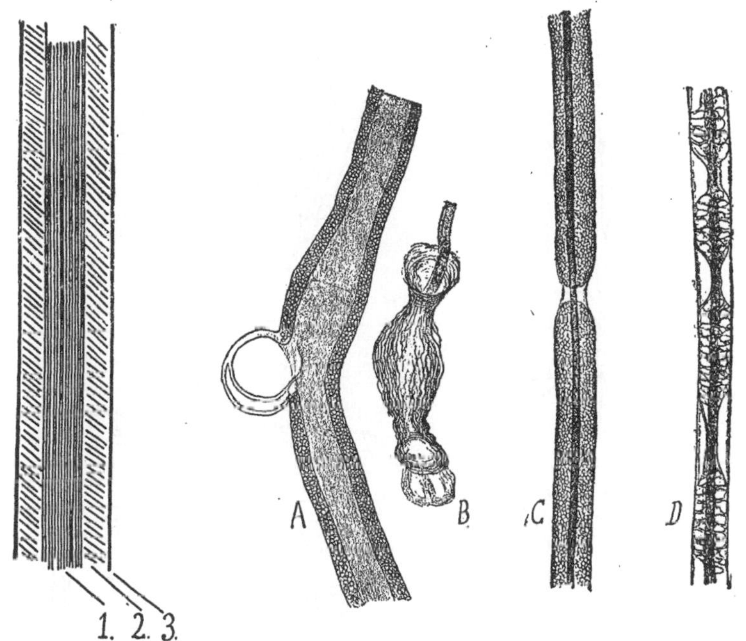

FIG. 24. Schematic sketch of a longitudinal section of a medullated neurone.

1 is the neurone itself (that is, a segment of the neuraxon).
2 is the medullary sheath.
3 is the sheath of Schwann.

FIG. 25. Drawings of (A) a section of a segment of a medullated neuraxon, and of (B, C, and D) the appearance of a medullated neuraxon, showing the structure and arrangement of the medullary sheath. After Kölliker, pages 10, 13 and 14, Figs. 331, 334 and 335.

And in the service performed by a neurone, although the whole cell is needed, the frayed-out ends and the fibres play the leading role.

Varieties of Neurones.—The cells that compose the nervous system vary tremendously in size and shape. They range from less than a twentieth of an inch to three feet or more in length. Some are very simple threads

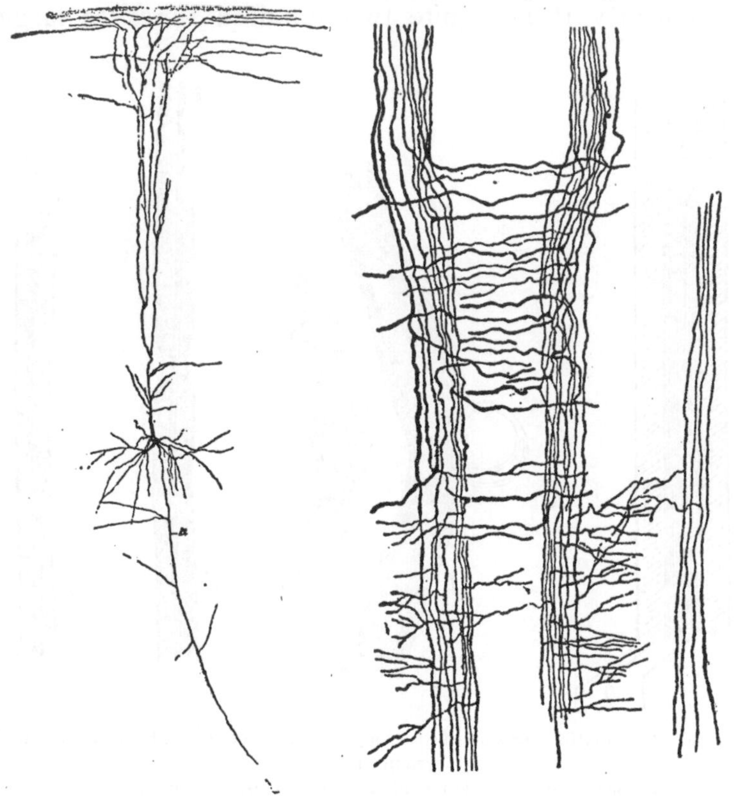

FIG. 30. A pyramidal neurone, showing only the beginning of the neuraxon. Greatly magnified. After Kölliker, 46, 367.

FIG 31. Segments of neurones with long neuraxons. Greatly magnified. After Van Gehuchten, II, 497, 676.

with a few frayings and side branches; others are at their two ends as complicated as the branches and roots of a tree. Some end in simple fibrils, others in discs or plates. These special forms are probably each adapted to the work the neurone has to do. With all these differences there remains the general likeness to a thread-like body frayed out at the ends, and along its course. Figs. 30-40, with those already given, show some of the chief types of neurone structure. They will serve also to emphasize the fact that the nervous system is made up of definite units.

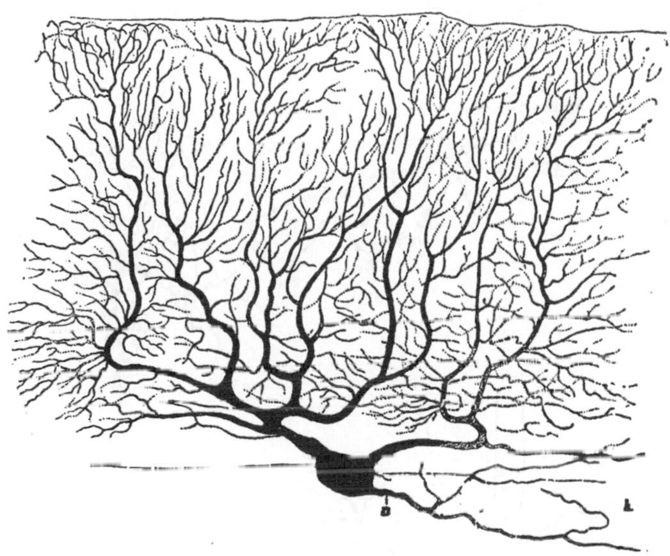

FIG. 32. A Purkinje cell, a type of neurone found in the cerebellum, characterized by very elaborate branching of the dendritic processes. Only a part of the neuraxon is shown. Greatly magnified. After Kölliker, 44, 363.

The Connections Between Neurones.—No neurone is in complete isolation. Every neurone stands in a special relation to one or more other neurones; namely, that some part of it is in close proximity or contact with some part of the other neurone or neurones. Probably it is between (1) the terminal arborization of the neuraxon or of one of its collaterals of one neurone and (2) the dendritic process or cell-body of the other that this close proximity obtains. I shall use the word connection to

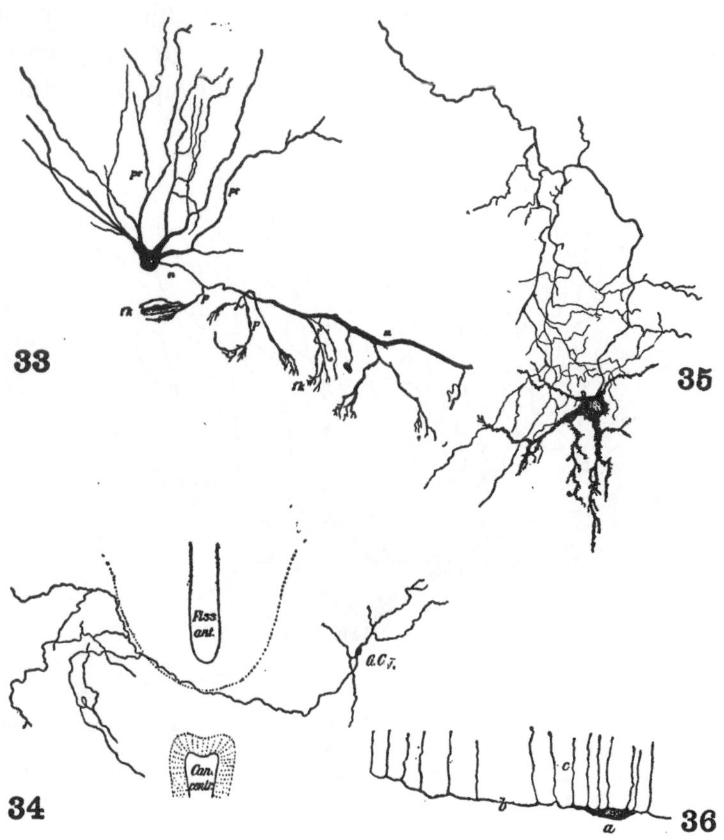

FIG. 33. A basket cell, a type of neurone found in the cerebellum. The neuraxon gives off a number of branches, each ending in a basket-shaped arborization. Greatly magnified. After Kölliker, 352, 535.

FIG. 34. A commissural cell, a type of neurone with a short neuraxon. Greatly magnified. After v. Lenhossék, 333, 50.

FIG. 35. A Golgi cell, a type of neurone with a short and much branching neuraxon. Greatly magnified. After v. Lenhossék, 371, 57.

FIG 36. A Cajal cell, a type of neurone with several neuraxons. Greatly magnified. After v. Lenhossék, 53, 8.

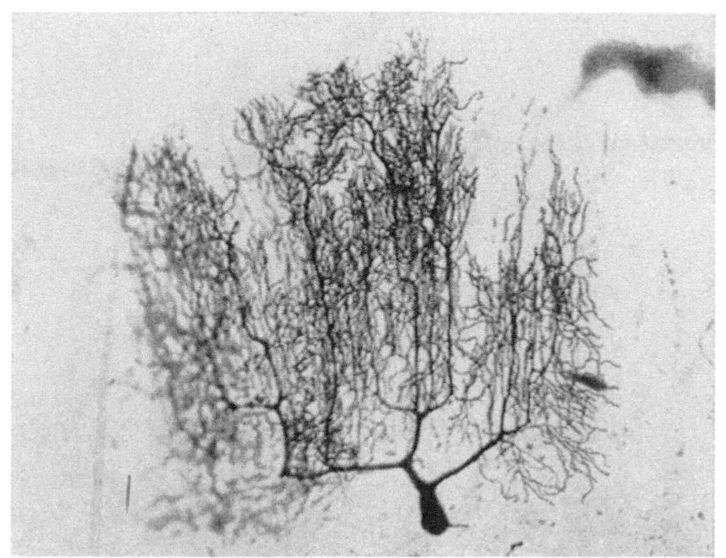

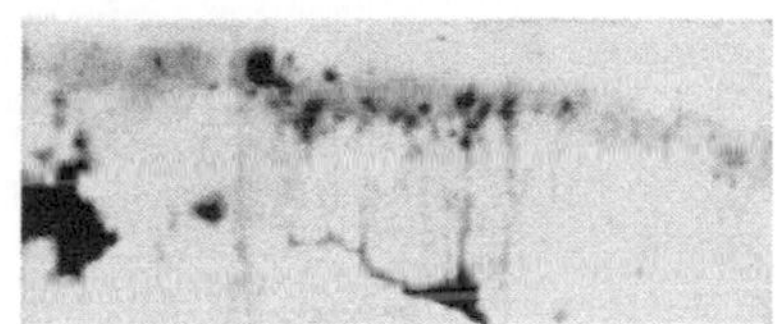

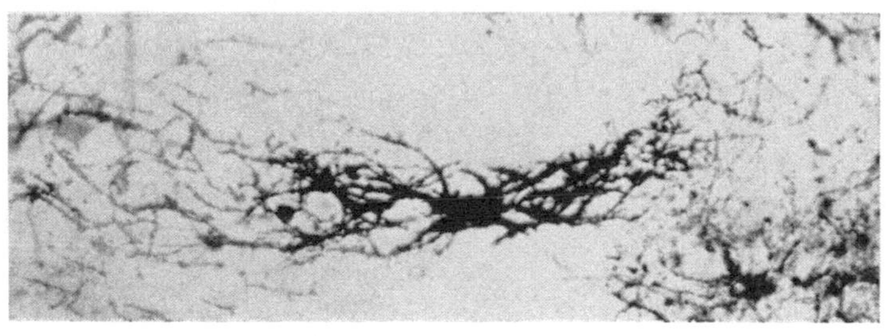

Fig. 38. A photograph of a Purkinje cell. After Starr, 35, Plate 15. ×125 Diameters.

Fig. 39. A photograph of a Cajal cell. After Starr, 65, Plate 37. ×125 Diameters.

Fig. 40. A photograph of a large polygonal neurone from the spinal cord. After Starr, 26, Plate 8. ×125 Diameters.

denote this relationship of close proximity or contact, though it should be understood that there may be, and commonly is, no connection in the sense of one neurone growing into the other, fusing with it, making a structural connection. Every neurone, then, is in connection[1]

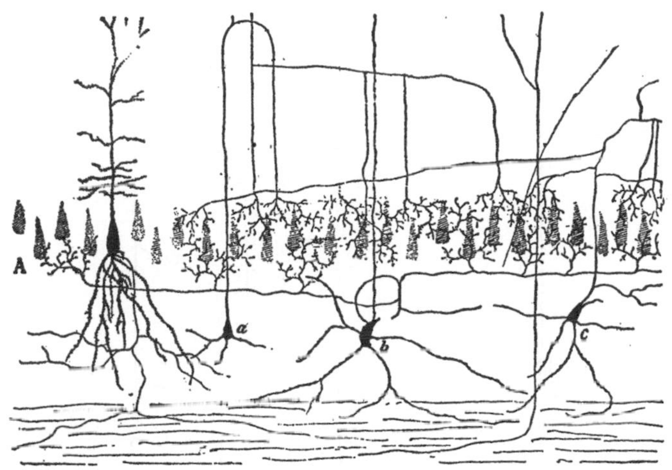

FIG. 37. Association cells (a, b and c). Greatly magnified. After Edinger, 28, 9.

with some other or others. Fig. 41 shows the general plan of such connections. Figs. 42 and 43 are drawings of the actual connections in two cases where they can be clearly inferred from what the microscope reveals.

[1] The word *synapsis*, meaning a clasping together, has been suggested as a useful descriptive term for the peculiar connections that exist between neurone and neurone.

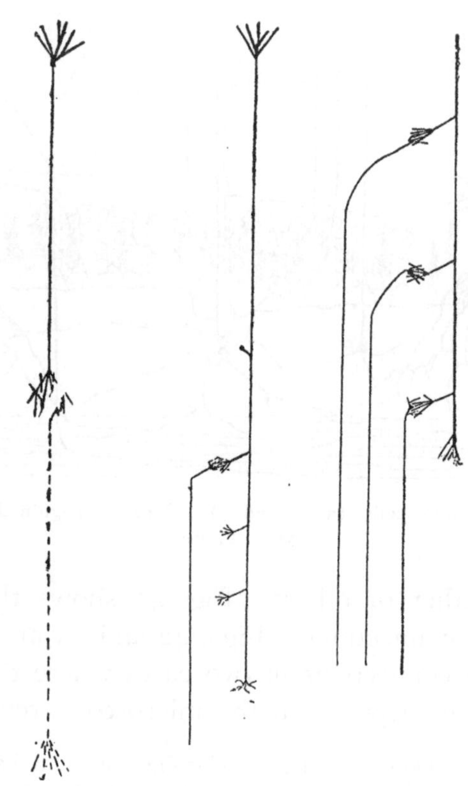

FIG. 41. A schematic sketch showing methods of connection between neurones.

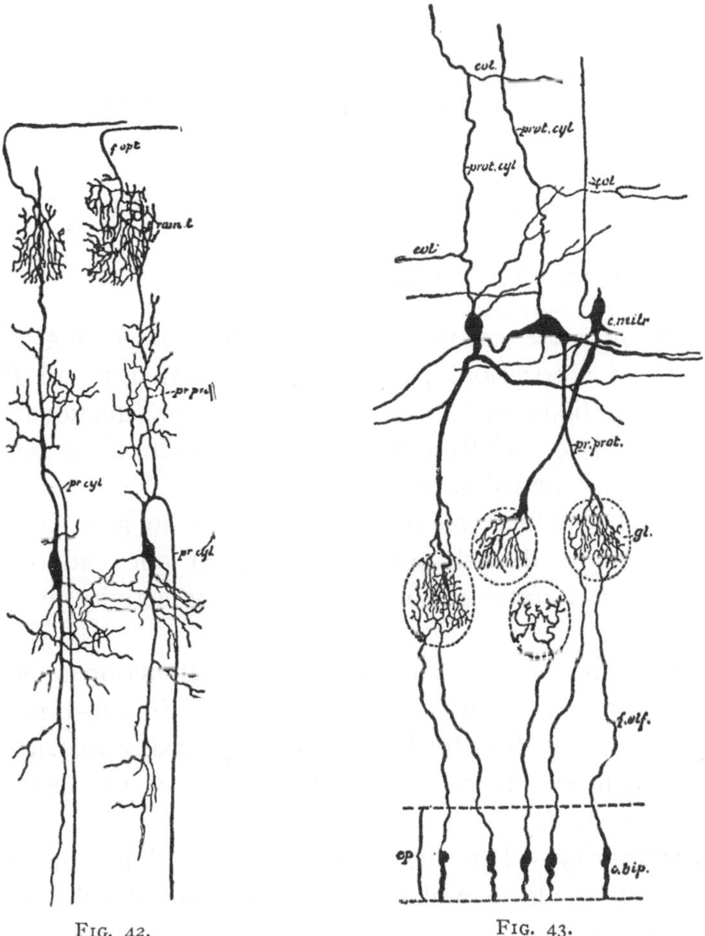

FIG. 42. FIG. 43.

FIG. 42. A sketch showing the connection between the terminal arborizations between the axis-cylinder processes of the neurones of the optic nerve and the dendritic processes of neurones in the optic lobes. f obt. = the axis-cylinder processes of the neurones of the optic nerve; ram. t. = their terminal arborizations in contact with the dendritic processes of the neurones below. After Van Gehuchten, I, 245, 159.

FIG. 43. A sketch showing the connection between the terminal arborizations of the bipolar neurones of the sense organ of smell and the dendritic processes of the so-called mitral cells. The two terminal arborizations intertwine in a globular mass called the glomerulus (gl). After Van Gehuchten, II, 369, 581.

CHAPTER X

The Action of the Nervous System

§ 25. *The Functions of the Neurones*

The neurone or nerve cell, besides possessing the powers of absorption, growth, etc., common to all the cells of the body, has three special duties or functions:—

(1) It is especially sensitive to or influenced by what happens to it or to parts of it.

(2) It conducts or transmits; *i.e.*, it so acts that a stimulation or disturbance or activity at one end of it results in a stimulation or disturbance or activity at the other.

(3) It is especially modifiable; *i.e.*, its action at any time depends upon its previous actions. In the human nervous system this third function is probably restricted in the main to the cells in certain parts of the central nervous system.

Sensitivity.—The first function, sensitivity or impressibility, needs no explanation. All matter is influenced by what happens to it; all living matter is especially so; and the nerve cells are the parts of living animals which carry this trait to the extreme. If we compare a man's body to a building, calling the steel frame-work his skeleton and the furnaces and power-station his digestive organs and lungs, the nervous system would include with other things the thermometers, heat regulators, electric buttons, door bells, valve openers,—the parts of the building in short which are specially designed to respond to influences of the environment.

Conductivity.—Just how the nerve cell conducts or transmits is not known. But the fact itself is sure. As a copper wire at one end of which an electric current is excited is so influenced that the current appears at the other end; as the air so acts that a vibration in any part spreads to other parts,—so the neurone when stimulated at one end acts so as to produce a corresponding activity at the other end; and so as to produce, under certain conditions, activity in the neurones in connection or synapsis with it.

The activity or disturbance which is transmitted is called the nervous impulse. When such an impulse is started in a nerve cell we say that the nerve cell is stimulated and call the agency by which the impulse is begotten the stimulus. Also when the nerve cell transmits the impulse to some body cells or other nerve cells we say that it stimulates them. Just as an electric current might pass along one wire, thence to another and along it to a third, so the nervous impulse passes from neurone to neurone when these are in functional connection.

The conduction or transmission is commonly over a series of nerve cells. For instance when the stimulus of pain at the finger's end makes us rub the injured spot, the impulse does not go from the skin to the muscles via a single cell (or set of cells), but traverses at least three, one set running from the skin to the spinal cord, one from the spinal cord to the muscles and one or more sets in the spinal cord connecting these. The transmission is, in any given neurone, usually, if not always, in the same direction; namely, toward the extremities of the neuraxon. A cell carrying impulses from the brain to a muscle does not, so to speak, carry return messages. For that another wire is used. A nerve cell may receive impulses from several nerve cells. It may and commonly does transmit its impulses to many nerve cells.

As might be expected, the two functions of sensitivity and conductivity are aided by such an arrangement of the nerve cells that stimuli are received at important points in the body and conducted to appropriate muscles. The constituents of the nervous system are not arranged at random. They are not like the chance tangle of a billion little threads which would receive stimuli hit or miss and conduct them nowhere in particular, but are, like the wires of the telephone system of a city or the railroads of a country, definitely placed lines of transmission between important points, and are so arranged at central offices as to permit a great number of useful connections. For instance, the neurones receiving the stimuli of light in the retina have definite connections with the neurones that carry impulses to the muscles that open and close the eyes, also to the muscles that move the eyes in turning to and converging upon and focussing for objects, also to the muscles that move the head.

Modifiability.—The analogy with a telephone system fails when we come to the third function, characteristic of many of the nerve cells[1] of the human brain, their power of modification by use. Unlike any system of wires or machines, the human nervous system possesses the power, at least in many of its parts, to be so altered by whatever happens to it as to enable the body on the next occasion to meet the situation more successfully. The nervous system which causes at a child's early sight of the fire the reaction of reaching for it, becomes a

[1]This paragraph refers only to the cells of the so-called 'higher' parts of the nervous system. Of the cells in the spinal cord and peripheral system it is almost surely not true. Of just what groups of cells it is true is not known.

nervous system that causes in later trials the reaction of avoidance. The connection between the impression and the one motor discharge has been weakened and an opposite one formed. The neurones learn, so to speak, to form, break and modify their inter-connections. If a telephone system possessed within itself the power by which the connections between the wires to certain houses would, with successful use, become more and more easily made while other connections would become increasingly more difficult, the analogy would be complete. But of course no mere machine has such a power to modify its workings, to make or break connections in accordance with the frequency of their use and the desirability or discomfort of the results to which they lead. This function of the neurones will be more fully described after the facts concerning the arrangement of the neurones in a system have been presented.

§ 26. *The Arrangement of the Neurones*

The Three Chief Groups.—The cells of the nervous system as a whole may best be divided into three classes. There are first, neurones which are stimulated by heat, light and other physical or chemical forces and discharge into other neurones; second, neurones which are stimulated by other neurones and themselves stimulate muscles; third, neurones which are stimulated by and themselves stimulate other neurones. In other words, there are cells directly sensitive to the environment, cells directly active in causing muscular contraction and cells acting as intermediaries between the former and the latter. The first are called *Afferent* or *Centripetal* neurones because they bring stimuli toward the brain and spinal cord (ad-fero= bring to); the second are called *Efferent* or *Centrifugal* neurones because they carry stimuli away from the brain and spinal cord toward the muscles. The third are called *Associative* or *Connecting* neurones.

Cells of class 1 are also called *Sensory* neurones or cells; cells of class 2, *Motor* neurones or cells. The term motor cell is also used to include cells which, though themselves not directly connected with muscles, lead out from the brain and connect in the spinal cord with cells which are so connected. Afferent, centripetal and sensory are used of nerves when the cells composing the nerve bring stimuli from the different parts of the body to the brain and spinal cord; efferent, centrifugal or motor nerves meaning of course nerves of an opposite function.

Sensory Neurones.—From almost every part of the body there originate afferent neurones to transmit stimuli arising there to the brain and spinal cord. Not only in the eyes, ears, nose, mouth and skin, but also in the muscles, articular surfaces, connective tissues, along the digestive tract, and throughout the sensitive areas of the body, there are neurone-endings capable of being set in action by the proper stimuli at the point where they are located.

Motor Neurones.—To all the muscles,—to the muscles which control the peristalsis of the intestine and the contraction of the blood vessels, as well as to those that more obviously move our limbs,—run efferent neurones, stimuli from which influence the amount and duration of muscular action.

The nervous system thus furnishes a most elaborate mechanism for receiving stimuli at almost all points in the body,—and, in the case of light, heat and smell, of stimuli from distant objects,—and for controlling the action of the body in the most minute details. If we liken the body to an army and the neurones to its signalling corps, we may say that signals may be sent from every point in the army to headquarters and from headquarters to every company or battery that can act.

Associative Neurones.—Still more elaborate is the mechanism for securing the proper connections between stimulus to and action of the body, for enabling the body to react advantageously with the movement fitted to the particular stimuli felt, for causing what happens to it to result in its doing what is necessary. This mechanism is of course the system of neurones connecting sensory with motor cells. It is almost literally true that any set of afferent cells may indirectly make connection with any set of motor cells and so influence any bodily act. The cell connections provide for a range of performances, extending from simple cases, such as that of the transmission of the stimulus of cells in the eye due to a bright light to the cells influencing the muscles of the eyes so as to result in the act of winking, to such a complex linkage as occurs when the sight of the word 'dollar' leads a man to put his hand in his pocket, grasp a coin and pull it out with a sigh.

The greater part of the bulk of the human brain is given up to such connecting cells. And the more important part of the work of the nervous system is the work, not of receiving stimuli from sensitive parts of the body, nor of discharging stimuli to the muscles, but of turning stimulus into discharge, connecting outgo properly with income, suiting expression to impression, action to circumstances.

The Grouping and Chaining Together of the Neurones.—It would be hopeless to try to portray in a diagram the arrangement of this practical infinitude of neurones to be affected by happenings inside and outside

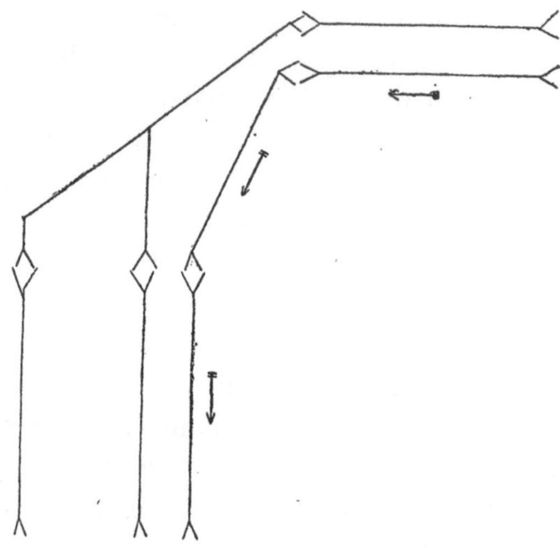

Fig. 44A. A possible scheme of arrangement of neurones to form an exceedingly simple nervous system.

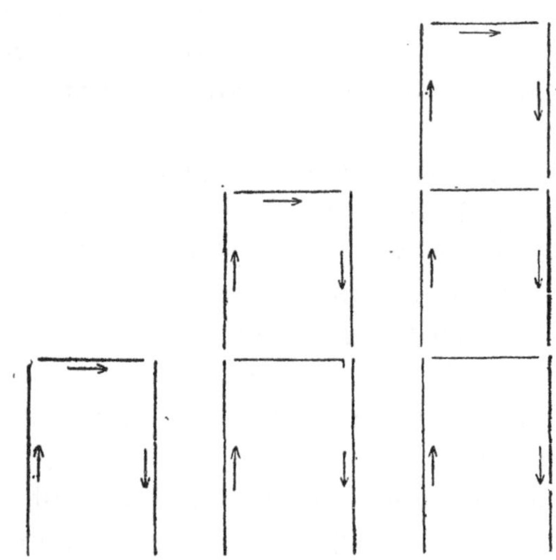

Fig. 44B. A scheme of arrangements of neurones of varying degrees of complexity. Each line represents one neurone or neurone group.

of the body and to transmit the stimuli here and there so as to make final connections with neurones going out to the muscles. Even if we knew the exact arrangement of each neurone in a man's brain it would take a model as large as St. Paul's Cathedral to make them visible to the naked eye, a model with whose details only years of study would familiarize us. Consider that counting at the rate of 50 a minute it would take a man working 12 hours a day over 200 years, probably over 700 years, to merely count the nerve-cells of one man.

It is possible, however, to picture the general features of the arrangement. We can imagine an animal with a nervous system with only two neurones to receive stimuli, only three neurones to discharge into muscles and only two connecting neurones. Fig. 44A may serve as its picture. Nervous action in general may be diagrammed as in Fig. 44B, which shows various degrees of complexity of connections. Even the most complicated nervous systems are variations of this general arrangement of a shorter or longer series of neurones making a circuit from sensitive surfaces to organs of response. Such a simple circuit is called a *Reflex arc* or *Reflex arch.* What would be seen if a perfect model of all the nerve cells were available would be simply a multitude of such arches or circuits of conduction from sensitive parts of the body to muscles and a multitude of circuits cross-connecting these.

It is possible also to get a more definite conception of these circuits of conduction by studying one or two samples or types of them. Figs. 45, 46 and 47 give in this way a general view of the grouping and chaining together of the neurones which conduct certain stimuli to the brain cortex or conduct stimuli from the cortex to certain groups of muscles.

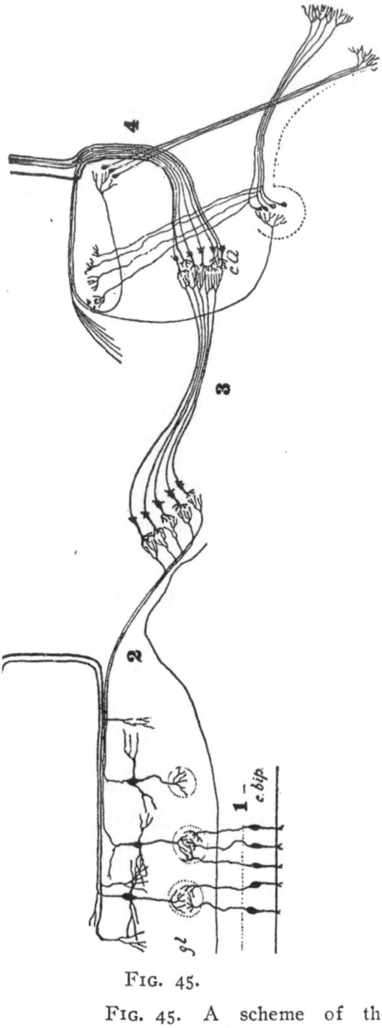

FIG. 45. 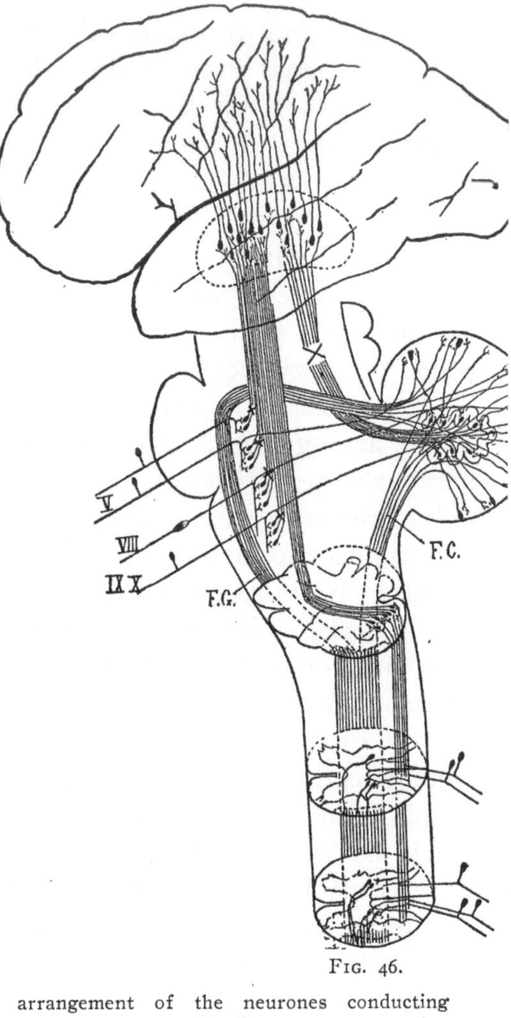 FIG. 46.

FIG. 45. A scheme of the arrangement of the neurones conducting stimuli from the olfactory sense organ. 1—the first neurones passing to the glomeruli (gl). 2—the second neurones passing from the glomeruli to the hippocampus. 3—the third neurones passing from the hippocampus to the cornu ammonis. 4—the fourth neurones passing from the cornu ammonis to make further connections. After Van Gehuchten, II, 294, 539.

FIG. 46. A scheme of the arrangement of the neurones conducting stimuli from the sense organs in the skin. After Van Gehuchten, II, 412, 624.

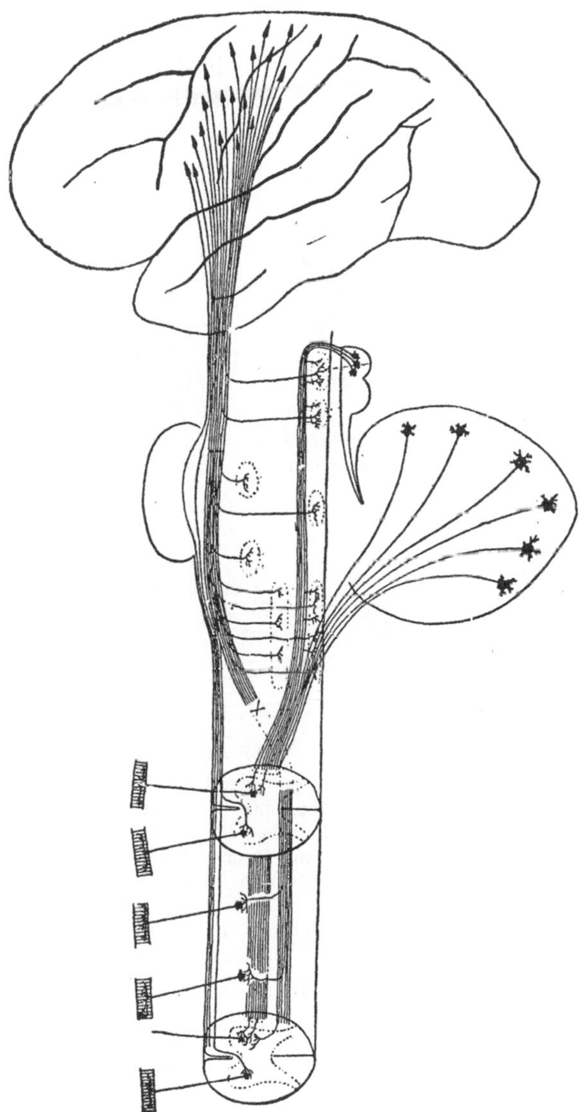

FIG. 47 Scheme of the arrangement of the motor neurones conducting stimuli toward the muscles. After Van Gehuchten, II, 512, 688.

Sense Organs.—One end (the peripheral end) of an afferent neurone is stimulated by physical or chemical forces. It may be more or less specialized to suit it to this work. It may be connected with bodily structures specially fitted to cause the physical or chemical force to influence it. The peripheral end of an afferent neurone, or a group of peripheral ends of afferent neurones which

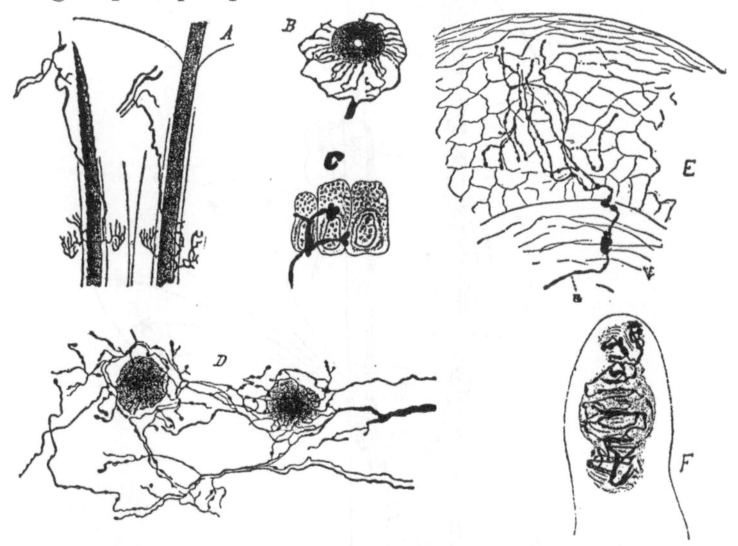

Fig. 48. A. Sensory neurones ending around the base of hairs (in the mouse). B. Cross-section of the same tissue as in A. C. Sensory neurones ending in epithelial cells. D. Sensory neurones ending around pigment cells. A, B, C and D are after Edinger, 42, 17. C is taken by Edinger from Bethe, D from Eberth and Bunge. E. Sensory nerve fibrils in the lining of the oesophagus. n—the neurone. After Barker, 362, 211; after Retzius. F. A sensory neurone's ending in a tactile corpuscle. After Barker, 386, 242; after Smirnow.

act as a unit, together with such bodily structures, is called a *Sense Organ.* A sense organ may be so simple an affair as the mere terminal arborization of a neurone ending freely in the outer or inner surface of the body. Such are shown in Fig. 48. It may be so complex as the eye, a sense organ which includes not only the endings of thousands of neurones in the retina, but also a lens to

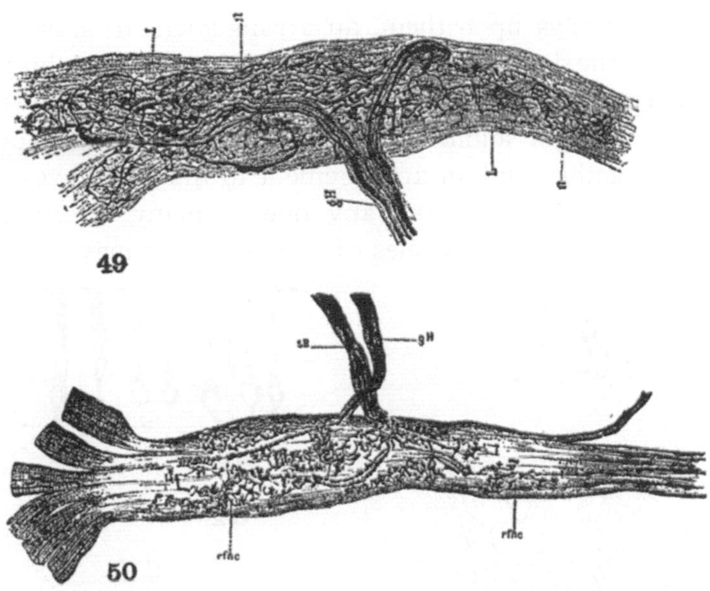

Fig. 49. Terminal corpuscle of Ruffini with the sensory neurone's ending therein. After Barker, 389, 246; after Ruffini.

Fig. 50. Tendon with nerve-plaque made up of the ending of sensory neurones seen entering from above; rfnc, ultimate arborization of the neurones. After Barker, 408, 266; after Ciaccio.

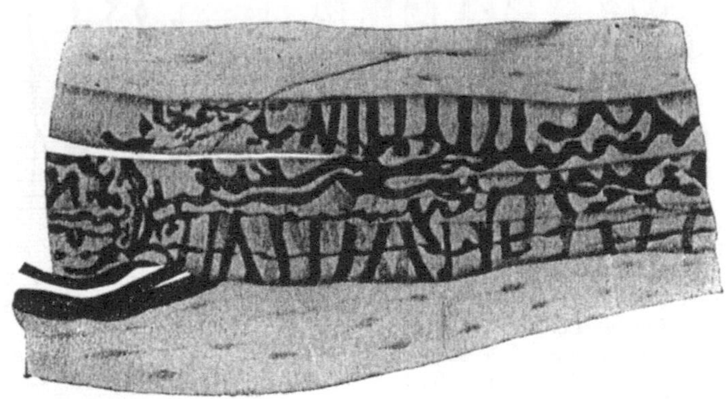

Fig. 51. Terminal plaque in a muscle spindle. The neurone entering at the left subdivides to form the elaborate net work shown. After Barker, 416, 273; after Ruffini

focus light rays upon them, an arrangement to alter the shape of the lens so as to focus the light from objects at different distances, an arrangement to regulate the amount of light admitted, an arrangement to shut out light altogether and an arrangement to move the eyes so that light will come from any one of many directions. The endings of the neurones of a sense organ may have a

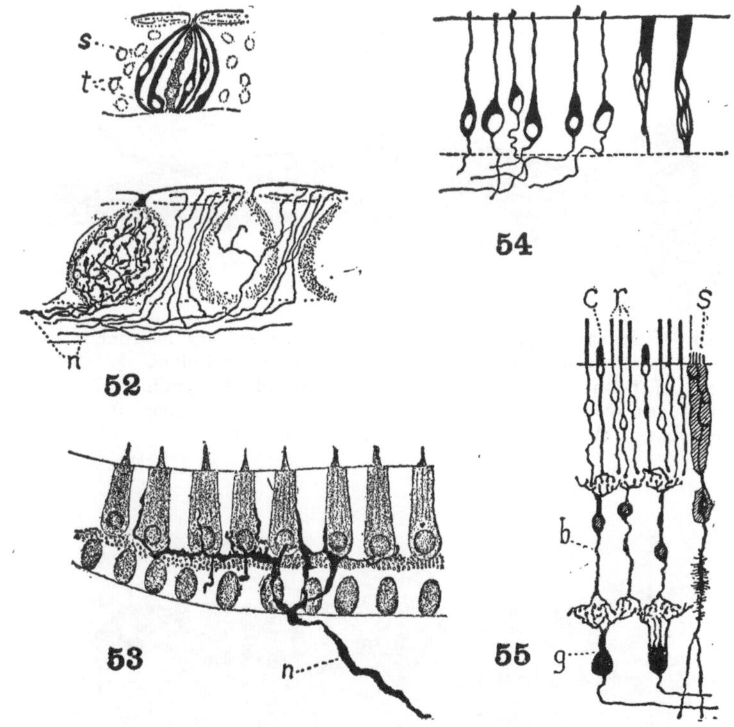

FIG. 52. Taste buds (from the tongue) and the endings of sensory gustatory neurones: s—a supporting cell; t—taste cells; n—fibrils of neurones passing upon and between the taste buds. After Barker, 527, 348; after v. Lenhossék.

FIG. 53. The ending of a sensory neurone in the ear (in the macula acustica sacculi). After Barker, 502, 333; after v. Lenhossék.

FIG. 54. Sensory neurones in the nose (in the olfactory mucous membrane). After Van Gehuchten, I, 244, 156.

FIG. 55. The principal nervous elements of the retina: r—rods; c—cones; s—a supporting cell; b—a bipolar nerve cell; g—ganglion nerve cell After Van Gehuchten, I, 244, 157.

structure not notably different from the general type (see Figs. 48, 52 and 53) or may be so altered as to be hardly recognizable (see Figs. 51, 54 and 55).

An adequate idea of the rich provision made in the nervous system for the reception of stimuli from without and within the body can be obtained only by study of such a full account of the peripheral neurones as may be found, say in Barker's 'Nervous System,' but Figs. 48-55 will give some conception of the fact and may serve to illustrate the statement previously made that "not only in the eyes, ears, nose, mouth and skin, but also in the muscles, articular surfaces, connective tissues, along the digestive tract, and throughout the sensitive areas of the body, there are neurone-endings capable of being set in action."

Motor Organs.—The ending of an efferent neurone in a muscle is specialized to suit its work of transmitting the nervous stimulus in some way to the tissue of the muscle so as to make the latter contract. As this process is almost, if not exactly, the same in all cases, there is not

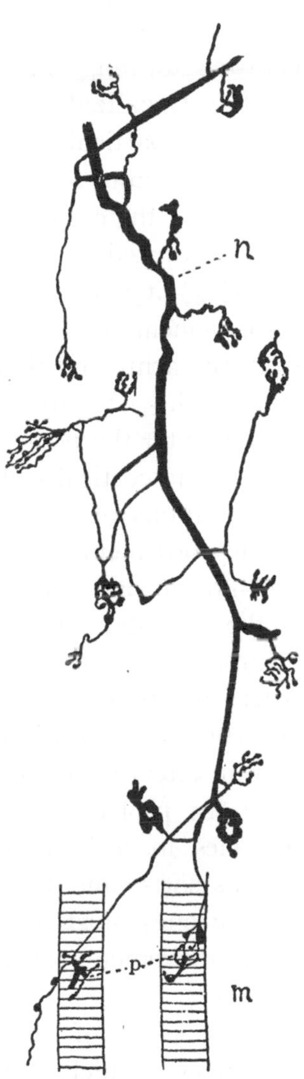

Fig. 56. The ending of a motor neurone in a muscle. At the bottom are shown two muscle plates (p) on muscle fibres (m). After Van Gehuchten, 242, 154.

the variety or complexity in motor organs which is found in sense organs. Fig. 56 shows the ending of a motor neurone forming the so-called *muscle-plates*.

The Localization of Brain Functions.—It is evident that each particular cell has its special work to do and that the circuits found at any particular spot in the brain have each their special work to do. If a man's spinal cord is injured in the lumbar region (the lower part of the back) it will not directly influence his feelings from or movements of his arms, since the cells that go to and from the arms and their connecting cells are not directly influenced. An injury to the frontal lobe does not directly alter the power of vision, for the circuit from the eyes to the cortical cells, action of which is accompanied by sensations of sight, is not impaired. But the section of the cord mentioned above would injure feelings from and movements of the legs. An injury at a certain spot in the occipital lobe would abolish sensations of sight. Injuries to the inferior frontal convolution result in disorders of speech. Injuries to the parietal region result in disordered sensations of bodily condition and secondarily in altered feelings of personality. Figs. 57 and 58 show the probable location in the human cortex of the neurones most intimately concerned with sensations of various sorts, and Figs. 59 and 60 show the location of the neurones most intimately concerned with the control of the movements of various muscles, in the case of the monkey.

This view of localization is quite different from phrenology, which regards the brain as divided sharply into parts each of which corresponds to some complex mental trait such as observation, ingenuity, kindness, intellect, attentiveness and the like. Such a complex trait as any one of these would involve very many differ-

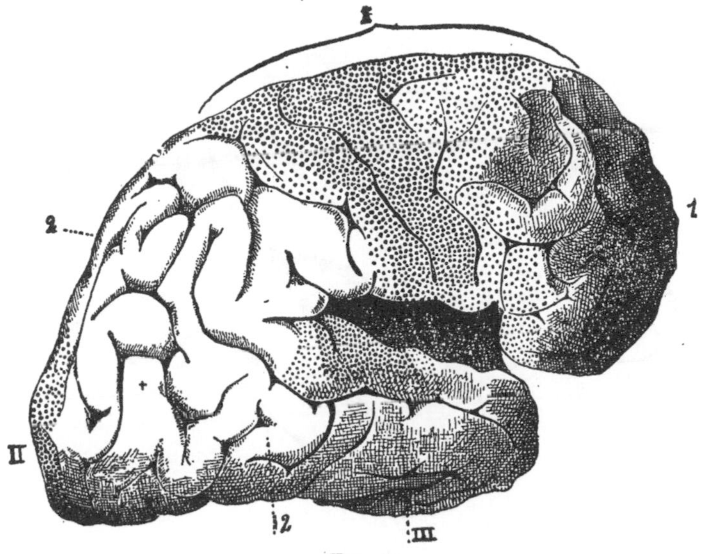

FIG. 57.

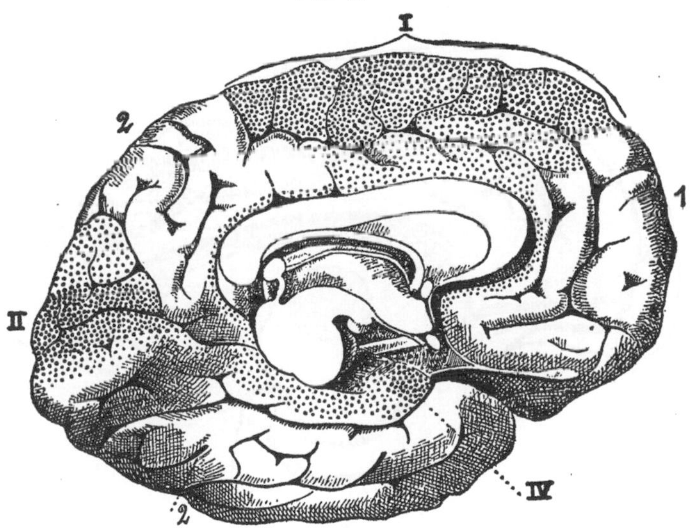

FIG. 58.

FIGS. 57 and 58. The areas of the cerebral cortex to which sensory neurones lead, and the areas occupied chiefly by associative neurones. FIG. 57 is a view of the outer half of the right cerebral hemisphere, FIG. 58 of its inner or mesial half. After Van Gehuchten, II, 308, 548; after Flechsig. I—Tactile area; II—Visual area; III—Auditory area; IV—Olfactory area. 1—Anterior area for association; 2—Posterior area for association.

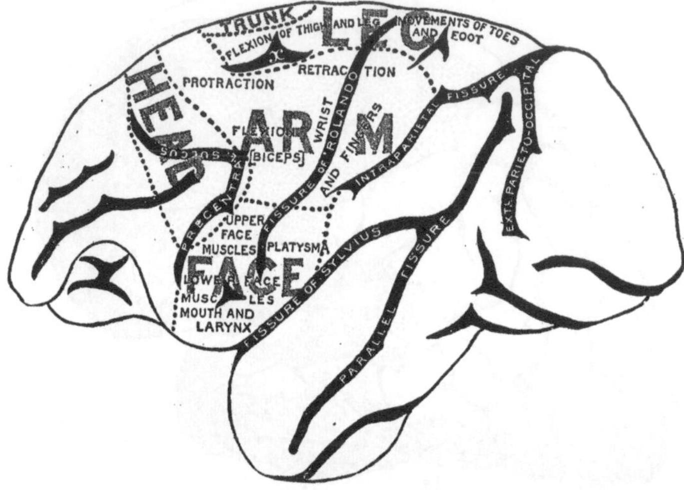

FIG. 59.

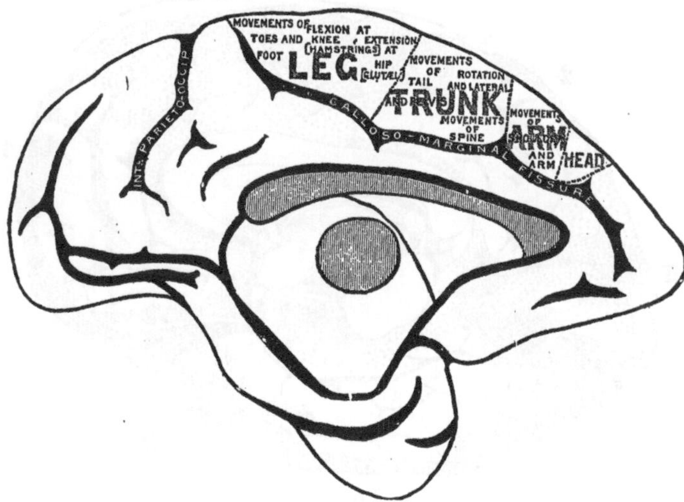

FIG. 60.

FIGS. 59 and 60. The areas of the cerebral cortex from which motor neurones stimulating certain movements lead (in the monkey). After Barker, 998 and 999, 634; after Horsley and Schaefer.

ent groups of neurones in many different parts of the brain. There is a place in the brain where the cells are specially connected with vision, but only the action of cells in many places would correspond to observation. Moreover 'place in the brain' means the entire course of a conducting group of neurones, or some important part of that course, not a compartment or special creative center.

The student should, therefore, not harbor any fanciful guesses, such as that each neurone corresponds to some one idea, or that one kind of a neurone goes with thought, another with emotions, or that the neurones hold thoughts and feelings in them or tied to them. The neurone is not a feeling, nor does it hold it, nor does the fact that the action of certain neurones is accompanied by, say sensations of smell, imply that the feeling of smell is in them.

The proper way to realize the nature of the human nervous system, the way its infinite multitude of nerve strings are arranged, the currents or stimuli which they transmit and the way these are aroused by happenings in the sense organs and in turn arouse movements of the body,—to realize in short the part played in human life by the nervous system—is to spend a year or more in the study of the histology and physiology of the brain. It is difficult from a few pages of words and diagrams to get even a general idea of what nerve cells are and what they do. If, however, the reader will practice himself in thinking at every sense impression, "Now a sense organ has been excited to action and has set up a commotion in some nerve cells. This commotion has been transmitted to other cells in the brain;"—if he will recall, whenever he makes a movement, that the movement is due to the contraction of certain muscles because of a stimulus transmitted to them by nerve cells running from the brain and spinal cord and ending in the muscle itself;—if he will, as he lives and thinks, keep before him an image of countless nerve cells running from this place to that in his brain and conducting impulses hither and yon, and think of this activity as the condition and parallel of his mental life;—if in short the reader will relate the facts so far given to his life of to-day and to-morrow, and think of human conduct in terms of the conduction of stimuli by nerve cells—he will come to realize and use the truth that the nervous system is the sum total of nerve cells, that these act by conducting impulses, that they link parts of the body that can be influenced to parts of the body that can act and link themselves to each other, that in the infinite number of their possible ways of conduction there is the basis and parallel of the infinite variety of a man's thoughts and deeds.

He will then no longer think of the nervous system as a vague name, but as an almost infinitely complex mechanism for receiving impressions from the body and its surroundings, for arousing and controlling bodily acts, for connecting the latter in appropriate ways with the various situations represented by the former, and for modifying their connections to meet the needs of life. He will realize the nature of the mechanism which enables us to respond to the events of our lives, and by its power of modification affords the physiological basis for changes of intellect and character, for learning, for education in the broadest sense.

§ 27. *The Laws of Brain Action*

The Law of Expression.—In accordance with the general doctrine of the conservation of energy we must believe that every stimulus that is started in sensory nerves by what happens at their peripheral ends must have some result. These stimuli cannot come to nothing. Their energy must either be transmitted on to other cells and eventually out through the efferent cells to the muscles, or else cause modifications,—do work,—in the cells of the central system. Just as in a storage battery electric charges coming in must sooner or later be discharged out or modify the battery itself, so the stimuli coming in to the brain must transform it or be conducted out and cause the muscles to contract. Every stimulus has its result somehow and somewhere. The function of mental life we saw was to influence our movements,—to cause what happened to us to result in actions that preserved our lives and happiness. The nervous system we now see to be a transformer of stimuli coming in, which are due to our surroundings, into stimuli going out which cause our actions, or into modifications of the nervous system itself.

Inhibitory Action.—That action in the nervous system discharges eventually into the muscles does not mean that it necessarily arouses movement. It may result in the cessation of a movement. Suppose that the forearm is being lowered by the contraction of the triceps and that a stimulus somewhere among the neurones works itself out into a stimulus to the biceps muscle. This stimulus tends to raise the forearm and, by counteracting or balancing the effect of the contraction of the triceps, may hold the arm still. Very many performances of skill require such a counteraction. Two sets of opposite muscles may both be stimulated, and but little movement be made. Twice as many neurones may be active as if the arm was swung energetically. Stimulation may regulate or decrease or check movement as well as initiate it. What we do *not do* as well as what we do, is often a result of stimulation. Every nervous impulse tends to work itself out in action, but action means restraint, the opposition of one contraction to others, not doing, as well as mere movement.

In the mental world as well, we may suppose that the action of the nervous system may be to check as well as to arouse a sensation or idea. Nervous action may make one *not* think of a certain thing, *not* feel a certain emotion.

When the result of nervous action is thus apparently negative,—when it checks or restrains or lessens,—the state of affairs is called *Inhibition* and the stimulus is said to inhibit the checked process. Such inhibitory action is of the utmost importance. We die when the vagus nerve to the heart is cut, not because the heart stops beating, but because it beats too fast; *i.e.*, over-acts. We are men and not brutes because the neurones concerned in the ideational and moral life keep in subjection and counteract the direct impulses to action of the neurones concerned in the instincts of greed, lust, cruelty and hatred. We reason, and do not merely day-dream, because we can check foolish, irrelevant fancies,—can inhibit all ideas that do not lead on to the desired goal.

The Law of Least Resistance.—When any neurone acts, *i.e.*, when it is stimulated and transmits, it will transmit the stimulus *along the line of least resistance*, or in other words along the line of strongest connection. Just as a copper wire through which an electric current is passing will, if its end is one millimeter from wire B and 20 millimeters from wire C, transmit the current to wire B, so a neurone will transmit its stimulus along the easiest path.

The line of least resistance or of strongest connection for any neurone or set of neurones will be, other things being equal, to the neurones which by the inborn arrangement of the nervous system are in closest connection with it. When the neurone endings of the retina are stimulated by bright light, nothing need happen in the leg muscles, because there is no ready made connection in the brain between the optic neurones and the neurones passing from the spinal cord to the leg muscles. But there will be a contraction of the muscles that lessen the pupillary opening, for there is a definite connection between the optic neurones and those to the iris muscle.

The Law of Inborn Connections.—The first law that decides what neurones any given neurone will arouse to action,—what the line of least resistance or strongest connection will be,—is then that, other things being equal, *any neurone group will discharge into the neurone group with which it is by the inner growth of the nervous system connected.* This we may call the *Law of Natural* or *Inborn Connections.*

The Law of Acquired Connections.—These natural lines of connection are in the course of life added to and subtracted from. The neurones are not by nature so arranged as to make a man say, "How dazzling," when the neurones of the retina are stimulated by a bright light. And the natural tendency of infants to turn the head toward a light is in later life largely overcome. The 'other things' are not always equal. We have in fact as a general law of behavior of, at least, the neurone groups of the so-called 'higher' centers or parts of the brain, the law that *when any neurone or neurone group is stimulated and transmits to or discharges into or connects with a second neurone or neurone group, it will, when later stimulated again in the same way, have an increased tendency to transmit to the same second neurone group as before, provided the act that resulted in the first instance brought a pleasant or at least indifferent mental state. If, on the contrary, the result in the first case was dis-*

comfort, the tendency to such transmission will be lessened.

In other words, *any conduction of a stimulus from nerve cell to nerve cell tends increasingly to take the direction it has taken unless the result is discomfort. In that case the original tendency decreases.*

Stating the law in terms of connections made between cells, we would say: *Connections between neurones are strengthened every time they are used with indifferent or pleasurable results and weakened every time they are used with resulting discomfort.*

This law includes the action of two factors, frequency and pleasurable result. It might be stated in a compound form as follows. (1) *The line of least resistance is, other things being equal, that resulting in the greatest satisfaction to the animal;* and (2) *the line of least resistance is, other things being equal, that oftenest traversed by the nervous impulse.* We may call (1) the *Law of Effect,* and (2) the *Law of Habit.*

The line of least resistance will also, other things being equal, be that most recently traversed. Suppose a neurone group, A, to have made connection ten times with neurone group B and ten times with neurone group C with equally pleasurable results; suppose the stimulus to have been transmitted from A to B ten years ago and from A to C during the past week. All that we know of living matter teaches us to expect that time will weaken the effect of any influence upon it. The strongest connection will then be from neurone group A to neurone group C. We may call this law the *Law of Recency.*

The line of least resistance will also be that which has been traversed by strong stimuli rather than weak, or by stimuli acting for a long time rather than by stimuli acting for a short time. Just as a large flow of water will cut a deeper channel than a small flow, or a flow lasting an hour a deeper channel than a flow lasting but a minute; so energetic or continued nervous transmission in a certain direction will make future transmission in that direction the more likely. We may call these the laws of *Intensity and Duration.*[1]

The line of least resistance will also be toward the most easily arousable, most sensitive neurone group, the group most ready to act.

All these different laws may be combined in the following general *Law of Acquired Brain Connections or Law of Association: When any neurone group, A, is stimulated, the nervous impulse will be transmitted to the neurone group which is most closely connected with group A, which has been aroused by A most frequently, with most satisfaction to the individual, most recently, most energetically and for the longest time, and which is the most sensitive at the time.*

Finally a neurone group may be, and commonly is, tremendously complex, and the connection formed may be, and often is, not with a few neurones, but with a few neurones chiefly plus a host of others acting less vigorously. The condition of a whole system of neurones at any one time determines their condition later. The action of any neurone group depends upon the 'set' or condition of the total system of which the group is a part.

The way in which a brain acts at any time is, then, the result of what connections it possesses as features of its inborn organization, plus what has happened to it in the past and what actions it has previously manifested.

[1]There is an important exception to the laws of frequency, recency, intensity and duration. If a connection is made *too* often, *too* energetically and *too* long *without rest,* the neurones may become fatigued and lose the power to transmit. Neurones, however, apparently fatigue very slowly.

From hour to hour and day to day it is becoming a new thing. From month to month it takes on new habits. Everything that is manifested as knowledge, power, self-control, habits of thought and action, attitudes and capacities of mind, skill and training may be paralleled within by alterations which the neurones have undergone. If we had perfect knowledge of the entire history of a man's brain, if we could from second to second see just what was going on in it, we should find in its actions and consequent changes the parallel of his life of thought and action.

Let no one object that it is incredible that the mental history of a man involving millions of ideas and acts should be paralleled by any bodily organ. A human nervous system is estimated to comprise over ten thousand millions of neurones. Each of these is itself a complex organ, and is often capable of many connections. Since it would take ten lifetimes to merely count the neurones and probably the lifetimes of ten Methuselahs to count their connections, it is evident that the brain is complicated enough to register the richest and most active human experience.

References

A. James, *Briefer Course,* VIII., IX.
Stout, *Manual,* 34-46.
Angell, *Psychology,* II.

B. Ebbinghaus, *Grundzüge,* §§ 7-11.
James, *Principles,* II., III.
Wundt, *Physiologische Psychologie,* II.-VI., or *Principles of Physiological Psychology,* II.-VI.
Barker, L. F., *The Nervous System.*

CHAPTER XI

The Nervous System and Mental States

§ 28. *In General*

Brain Action Without Consciousness.—Not all the happenings in all the neurones are accompanied by mental states. Stimuli are incessantly coming in from the body which need not be felt; *e.g.*, many stimuli from the lungs or digestive tract in waking hours; many stimuli from all quarters during sleep; many stimuli of slight amount. Stimuli are incessantly going out to the muscles which some psychologists think are never felt and which certainly in many cases and at many times are not; *e.g.*, the stimuli which regulate the nourishment of parts of the body and control the reflexes such as winking or the contraction of the pupil of the eye.

Brain Action With Consciousness.—What sort of action in the neurones is accompanied by consciousness and even whether there is any special sort that is, science has not yet discovered. Which neurones are concerned in the conscious life is known only imperfectly. Apparently in man those in certain parts of the cortex are and those in the sensory and motor nerves, spinal cord, medulla, cerebellum and base of the brain are not. It is thought by many that consciousness appears only when the nervous system is undergoing modification,—becoming adjusted to some new condition.

The action in the nervous system which is connected

with any mental state is called the physiological or neural or nervous basis or correlate of that mental state.

Although it is easy to prove that mental life *in general* is connected with the activity of nerve-cells it is hard to ascertain what is the *particular* physiological basis of each special variety of mental state. For instance, just what happens in the nervous system when one feels bored or thinks 'nevertheless,' no one could say. So also what difference there is between the neural correlate of the mental image of a dog and the neural correlate of a general notion of a dog is a matter for hypothesis, not for proof.

There are undoubtedly differences in the activities of the nervous system corresponding to the differences between feelings. For sensations there is brain action A, for percepts, brain action B, for images, brain action C, for emotions, brain action D, and so on through the list. With the advance of knowledge these correspondences will become better and better known. In some cases there is already enough evidence to warrant a working belief. In others there are more or less interesting hypotheses. These beliefs and hypotheses are stated briefly in § 29.

§ 29. *The Physiological Correlates of Particular Groups of Mental States*

Of Sensations.—The physiological basis of a sensation is action of certain neurones stimulated at the time by sensory neurones. The locality in the brain of the neurones concerned in many special kinds of sensations, *e.g.*, sounds, is known. In Figs. 57 and 58 were shown the localities in the brain where the neurones concerned with certain sensations are found. It is not action of sensory neurones themselves, of the cells making up the afferent nerves, that parallels sensations. It is apparently only when the afferent cells have stimulated other cells than themselves, cells in the cortex of the brain, that any sensation is felt.

Of Percepts.—The physiological basis of a percept is the same except that modifications of the action of the neurone group due to previous experiences play a larger part. It is apparently when the actions of neurones stimulated by sensory neurones result together in some unitary muscular response that we feel, not a confusion of sensations, but a definite 'thing.'

Of Illusions and Hallucinations.—The physiological basis of an illusion is the same as for the corresponding percept except that the sensory neurones that give the stimulus are not those which commonly do. The physiological basis of an hallucination is the same as for the

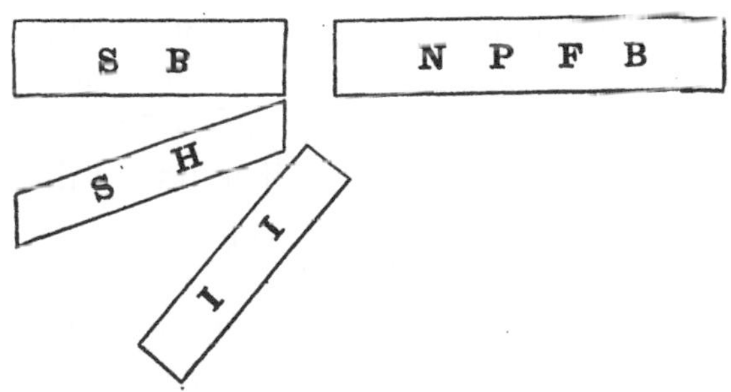

FIG. 61. Let N P F B be the neural process corresponding to the feeling of the sound of a bell. Let S B be the action in sensory neurones which usually arouses the neural process corresponding to the feeling of the sound of a bell. Let S H be the action in sensory neurones which usually arouses the neural process corresponding to the feeling of the sound of a hammer on an anvil. Let I I be the neural process corresponding to the feeling of certain ideas and images. When S B arouses N P F B, the mental state corresponding is called perception. When S H arouses N P F B, the mental state corresponding is called illusion. When I I arouses N P F B, the mental state corresponding is called hallucination.

corresponding percept except that the cells are aroused to action without any stimulus from sensory cells. Fig. 61 illustrates the different neural processes which parallel respectively the percept, illusion and hallucination of an object.

Of the Emotions.—With respect to the coarser or bodily emotions such as jealousy, rage or fear, the best working hypothesis is the theory[1] that their physiological basis is, like that of sensations, the action of neurones stimulated at the time by afferent neurones. In the case of the emotions, however, these afferent neurones come, not from eyes or nose or ears, but from the lungs, heart, blood vessels and other internal organs.

That is, just as when, light rays having excited the peripheral ends of the visual sensory neurones, the excitation is transmitted to the sensory neurones concerned in vision, sensations of color and brightness are felt; so when the excitation caused in the peripheral ends of the sensory neurones in the internal organs of the body by palpitating heart, tense muscles, the contraction of the small arteries of the skin, etc., is transmitted to the neurones in the cortex, fear is felt. The bodily disturbances which are commonly called the expression of the emotional feeling would then be really its cause. The tremendous equipment of sensory neurone endings in the inner parts of the body appears to be not so much for the sake of the few sensations such as hunger, thirst, nausea, pains and the like which are recognized as dependent upon afferent neurones from inside the body, as for the sake of the rich life of passion, jealousy, fear, anger, grief, joy and the like.

[1] The James-Lange theory of the emotions, named after the two psychologists, William James and C. Lange, who announced the theory independently at about the same time.

According to the other theory of the emotions, the physiological basis of the emotions would be the action of associative neurones aroused by the neurones the action of which parallels percepts and ideas. By this theory the order of events is (1) some sensation, percept or idea, (2) some emotion resulting from it, (3) disturbances of bodily organs resulting from the emotion. The behavior of a child frightened by, say, a horse would be described by the two theories as follows:—

Older Theory	*James-Lange Theory*
Percept of horse running.	Percept of horse running.
Feeling of fear.	Acts of altered heart beat, pallor, trembling, etc.
Acts of altered heart beat, pallor, trembling, etc.	Feeling of fear.

The two theories might be stated in terms of neurone action as follows:—

Older Theory	*James-Lange Theory*
Sense organs stimulated.	Same
Afferent neurones.	Same.
Central neurones concerned with percepts.	Same.
Central neurones connected therewith (giving the emotion).	Motor neurones.
	Bodily disturbances in heart, lungs, etc.
Motor neurones.	Afferent neurones coming from heart, lungs, etc.
Bodily disturbances in heart, lungs, etc.	Central neurones connected with these (giving the emotion).

It is a matter of dispute how far other than the coarser of emotions follow the James-Lange theory. It appears probable that the bulk of our emotional life is thus due to stimuli from the heart, lungs, vaso-motor system, digestive tract and other internal organs; that in large measure the emotions are caused in the same way as sensations and percepts,—are 'peripherally initiated' mental states. There still might be and probably are not only such sensory emotions but also imaged emotions, 'centrally initiated.' Their neural correlates would correspond to those for images of things, to be described on the next page.

Of Effort.—The physiological basis for the feeling of strain or effort, as in voluntary attention, also corresponds probably to that for sensations, being action of certain neurones stimulated at the time by sensory neurones with peripheral ends in or on the muscles, joints and tendons.

Of External Relationships.—Feelings of external relationships, such as of above, below, beyond and the like, may be really sensational; *e.g.*, the feeling of the aboveness of this line to the next may be simply the feeling of the eye's movement in looking from one to the other. The neural correlate of feelings of relationship of this sort would be the same as of sensations.

It may perhaps be assumed that all the feelings which were grouped under the heading, *feelings of the first intention,* have as their neural correlate action in neurones stimulated at the time by afferent neurones.

Leaving now the field of sensations and their like, all statements about neural correlates of mental states must be regarded as hypotheses and should properly be prefaced by a perhaps.

Of Images.—The neural basis of feelings of the second intention is evidently action of cells *not* stimulated at the time by sensory cells. Much more cannot be said except as guess work. The physiological basis of an image is perhaps action similar to that in the corresponding percept but weaker, or (and to the author's mind far more probably) the action of only a portion of the cells involved in the corresponding percept, the cells associated in the action being different in the two cases. In actual perception the brain action giving, say, the mere sight of the thing would be accompanied by brain action corresponding to the thing being in a certain place, being touched as well as seen, being felt as possessed of tendencies to be or do this or that. The neural correlate of a percept, say of a dog, would thus be a complex total. The mental image of the dog might well have as its neural correlate a weakened revival and of only a part of this total.

Still more hypothetical are all notions about the neural correlates of feelings of the third intention.

Of General Notions.—The physiological basis of a general notion is perhaps the neural correlate of some percept or image or sensation, commonly of a word, plus the half-aroused activities of the numerous associated sets of cells, each set of which would, if fully active, give the feeling of one of the particular things included in the class meant by the word. For instance, the concept 'a dog' would have as its physiological basis the cell action going with the image of the word 'dog' plus the half-aroused action of the cells which if fully active would give images of different particular dogs.

Of Individual Notions.—The physiological basis of an individual notion is probably the neural correlate of some percept or image or sensation, commonly of a word, plus action in other cells which would, if allowed to discharge on into their associated cells, lead to the image or percept of the thing or person referred to by the individual notion. Thus the thought of 'Napoleon' may have as its physiological basis the cell action going with the word 'Napoleon' plus the half-aroused action of the cells which if fully active would give images of Napoleon or of his various acts and characteristics.

Of Feelings of Relationships.—Feelings of logical relationships may have as their basis the states of transition in the brain from the activity of one set of neurones to that of others. For instance, the feeling of unlikeness may have as its parallel the simultaneous waning of one brain process and the waxing of one different. Some feelings of relationship may be semi-emotional feelings, and due to the same type of neural action as parallels emotions. Thus the feeling of the relation of cause and effect may be a feeling of justified expectancy.

Other hypotheses about the neural basis of mental states are that the greater or less intensity of a mental state is due to a greater or less violence of the conducted stimulus; that the personal feeling which characterizes mental states is related to the constantly acting cells stimulated by ever present bodily conditions; that the broad qualities of mental life which we call temperament or disposition are related to cell action due to the condition of the blood. About the physiological activities which go with feelings of time, belief, desire, choice and many other types of feelings, so little is known or even guessed that it is unwise to note the speculations about them.

Of Mental Connections.—The physiological basis of the *connections* between ideas, acts, and ideas and acts is much clearer than the physiological basis of the varieties of ideas. These connections are throughout based on the connections between neurone and neurone in the nervous system, the existence of paths of easy conduction for the nervous stimulus.

Reflexes and instincts are the manifestations in conduct of connections between neurones due to the natural organization of the human body. Acquired habits of thought and conduct represent the connections between neurones by which the nervous system has adapted itself to the individual's needs. When in Part III the growth of mental life and the laws of its action are described, the dependence of the connections between the parts of a human life of thought and action upon the connections between parts of the nervous system will be seen everywhere to be a natural, almost the inevitable, conclusion.

Exercises

Experience 13. The Influence of the Absence of Neurone Endings in a Portion of a Sensitive Surface. The neurones composing the optic nerve form a compact bundle of fibres where they enter the retina. Where this bundle enters there are no rods or cones or bi-polar neurones, nothing in fact to be stimulated by light.

Close or cover the left eye. Look with the right eye steadily at the cross in Fig. 62. When the book is about seven inches from

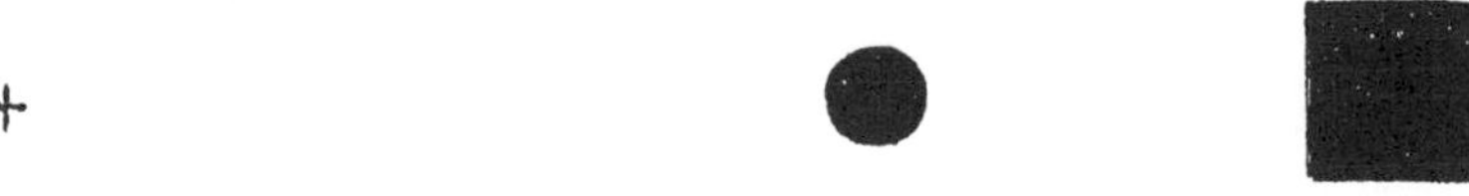

Fig. 62.

the eye the circle will not be seen at all. It is essential that the eye be kept fixed steadily on the cross. The reason for the non-appearance of the circle is that at that distance the image of the circle on the retina falls on the spot where the optic nerve enters. Move the book slowly to a greater distance, fixating the cross as before. Soon the circle will reappear and the square dis-

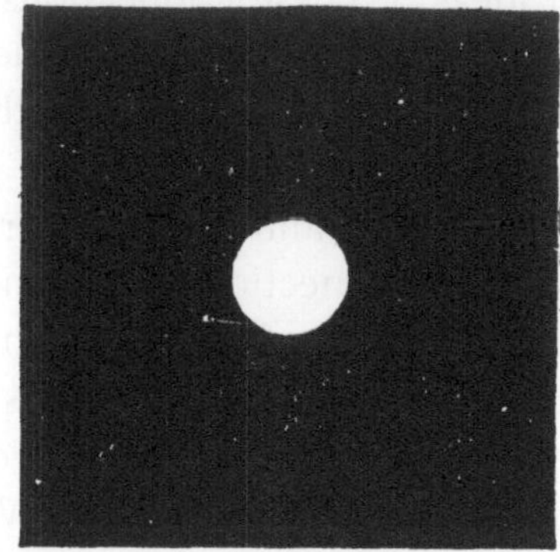

FIG. 63.

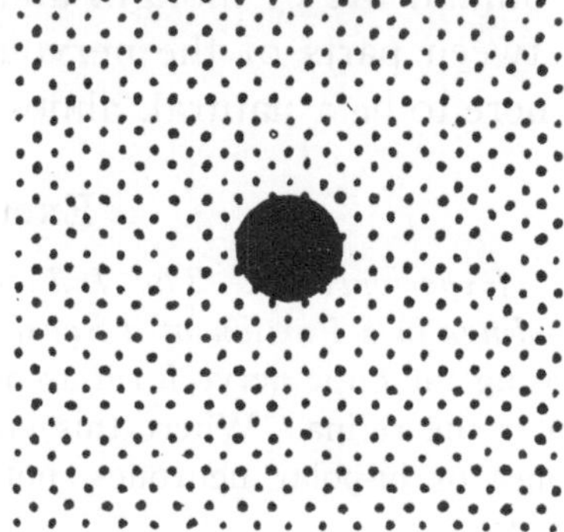

FIG. 64.

After some time, I came thither dressed in my new habit, and now I was called governor again. Being all met, and the captain with me, I caused the men to be brought before me, and I told them I had had a full account of their villainous behaviour to the captain, and how they had run away with the ship, and were preparing *° ^ommit further robberies; but that .ce had eusnared them in their ow d that they were fallen into the pi ey had digged for others. I let them , that by my direction the ship had been seized, that she lay now in the road, and they might see by and bye that their new captain had received the reward of his villainy; for that they might see him hanging at the yard-arm. That as to them, I wanted to know what they had to say, why I should not execute them as pirates taken in the fact, as by my commission they could not doubt I had authority to do. One

FIG. 65

appear. Why? How may the figure be used to demonstrate the existence of the similar 'blind spot' in the left eye?

From this experiment it would appear that every field of view seen by a single eye should have an unseen spot or patch.

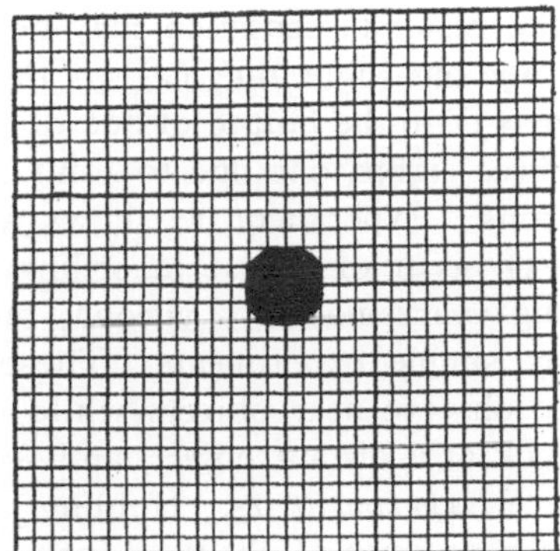

Fig. 66.

Perform a similar experiment with Figs. 63, 64, 65, 66 and 67. When the circle falls on the blind spot, what takes its place in each case? State the rule which seems to hold concerning what happens (in the case of vision) in the absence of neurone endings in a portion of a sensory surface.

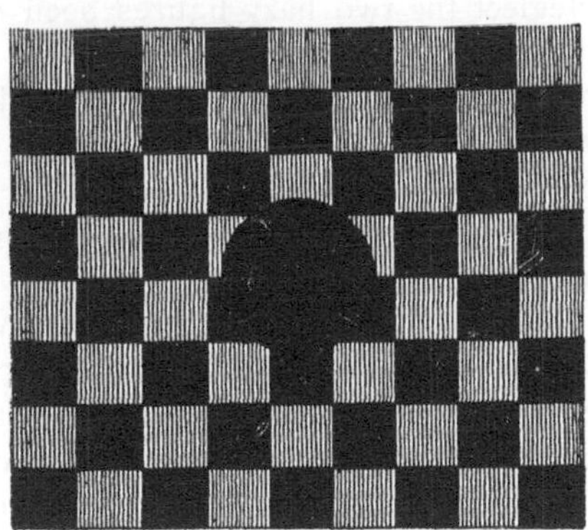

Fig. 67.

Sensations from Bilaterally Symmetrical Sensitive Surfaces.

Experiment 14. If you touch the desk simultaneously with the right and left forefingers, you feel two touches, but if you hear a bell with both ears or see a star with both eyes you ordinarily feel but one sound or star. Recall and perform the experiment familiar to childhood by which the eyes are made to see double.

In binocular vision each retina is separately stimulated, but the result in sensation may be (1) two corresponding sights, or only one sight due (2) to the joint action of the two stimuli or (3) to the failure of one of them to influence sensation, or (4) three sights, one due to joint action and two to the separate actions. Experiment 14 shows a case of (1). Cases of (2) and (3) occur of course in ordinary life (cases of 2 occurring during every moment's vision), but they may be seen most clearly by simple experiments. These experiments involve the power to observe near objects while holding the eyes as one would to look at a distant object, and so may require a little practice.

Experiment 15. Holding the book upright before the eyes at a distance of about 12 inches, look at the drawings of Fig. 68 as you would to look through it at an object in the distance. That is, fixate for a point in the distance, so that the left eye looks at the left hand pair of circles and the right eye at the right hand pair. If this is done the two figures will appear to move toward each other and occupy the same space. If the eyes are kept as if fixed on a distant object, the single figure resulting from the two drawings can be kept in place for examination. Neglect the two hazy figures seen one on each side of it. What does it appear to be? What new feature not present in either of the two figures appears? Do likewise with Fig. 69. Fill out with appropriate words the blanks in the following statement:— In certain cases when one retina receives one impression and the other another impression, the resulting percept is of........, and possesses the quality of ....

Perform the same experiment with Fig. 70. What is the resulting single percept? Do the bars of the cage hide part of the bird or does it hide part of the cage? Does it seem inside or outside or against the front of the cage?

Experiment 16. Combine the two halves of Fig. 71 by fixating for a point in the distance as in Experiment 15. What is the resulting picture? Hold it steadily for some moments. What happens?

Do likewise with the two drawings of Fig. 72.

Do likewise with the two drawings of Fig. 73.

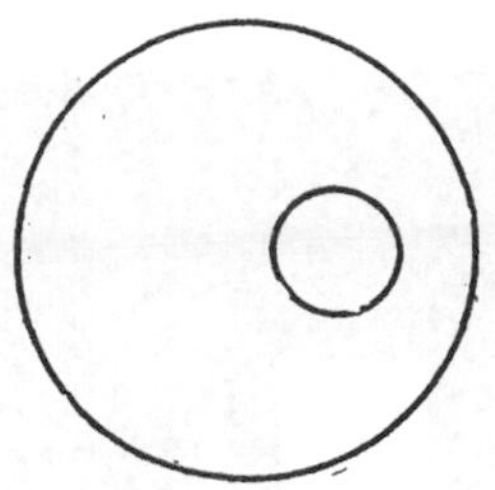

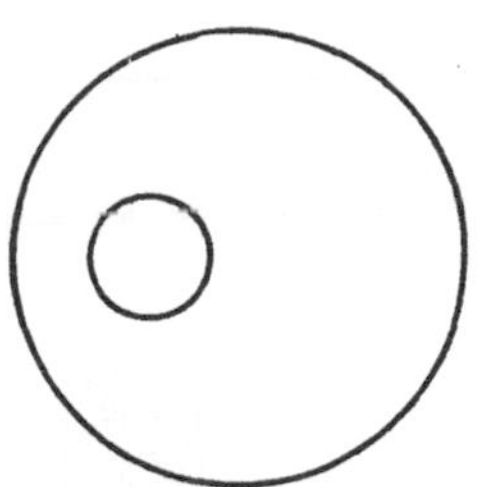

Fig. 68.

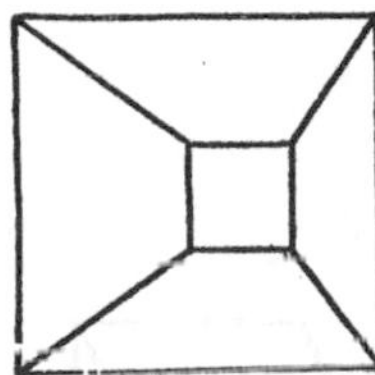

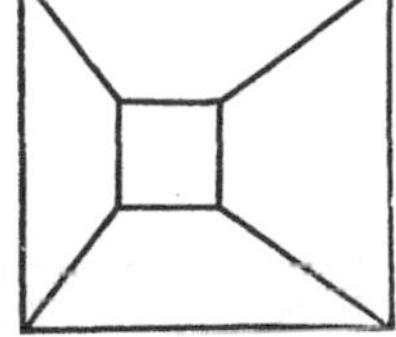

Fig. 69.

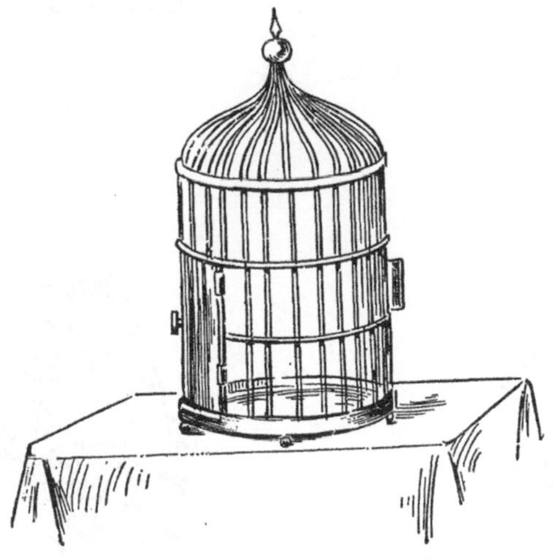

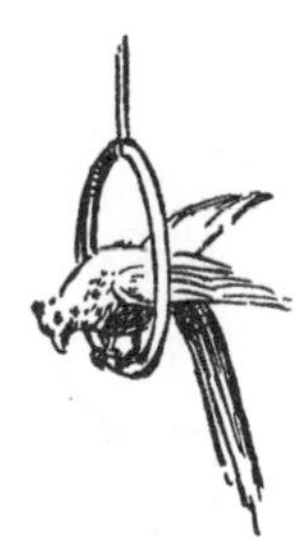

Fig. 70.

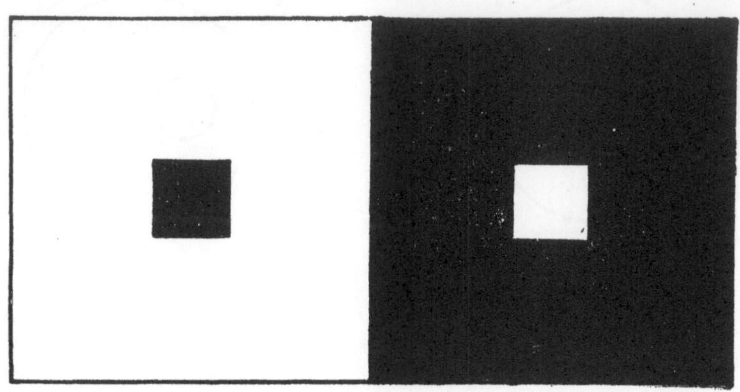

FIG. 71.

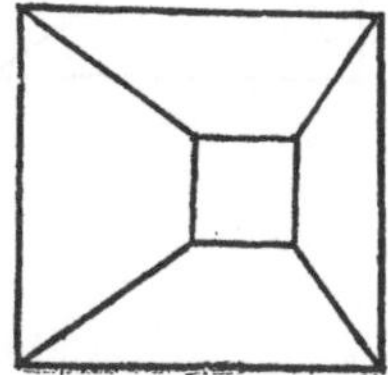

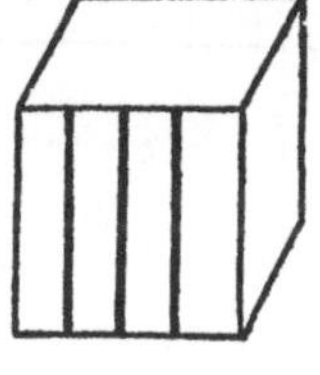

FIG. 72.

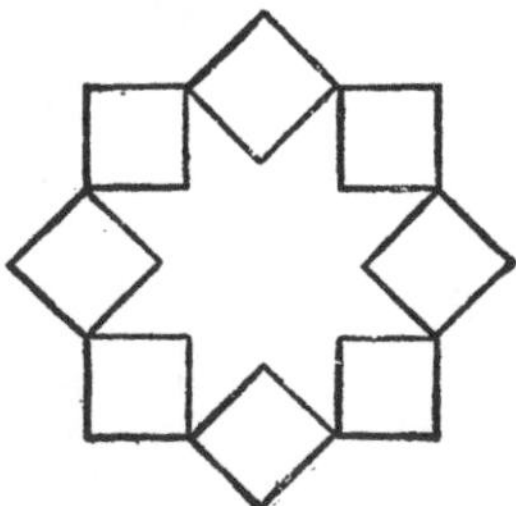

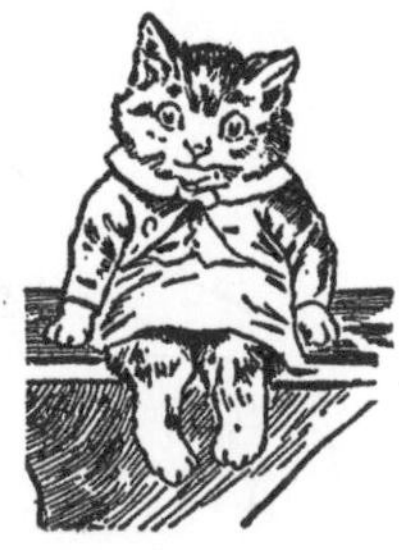

FIG 73.

What is the chief difference between the resulting percepts in Experiment 15 and those in Experiment 16? What are some other differences? What difference between the pairs of objects of Figs. 68-70 and the pairs of objects of Figs. 71-73 seems to account for the difference in the resulting percepts? Fill out with appropriate words the blanks in the following statement: Two differing retinal impressions will result in a single and constant percept if they are the impressions which would ordinarily be caused by ...., or are .... such impressions. They will result in .... if they are impressions which could not be caused by ....

References

A. James, *Briefer Course,* II. (9-12), III. (28-40), IV. (47-53), V. (60-67), XIII. (228-234), XIX. (310-311), XX. (329-330) XXIV. (375-384).

Angell, *Psychology,* III.; see also pp. 93-101, 137, 190-192, 215f., 272f., 316-319.

B. James, *Principles,* XI. (434-447), XVI. (653-658), XVII. (68-75), XIX. (103-106), XX. (449-474.)

PART III

DYNAMIC PSYCHOLOGY

§ 30. *Introduction*

The previous chapters have described the different varieties of mental states, the service performed by each in the conduct of life, and the physiological facts with which they are connected. Equally important—for practical purposes more so—is knowledge of the mind in action, knowledge, that is, of the facts and laws which determine what any human being will think and feel and do, how he will learn, why he will misunderstand, when he will be interested, what habits he will form, to what sort of intellect and character he will attain. The science of the mind in action is called **Dynamic Psychology.**[1]

If we ask how the baby comes to feel pleasure at pulling and overturning a toy, why we shut our eyes when an object approaches them, or why we feel the sun to be brighter than the moon, common experience readily answers that we are by nature provided with these and other tendencies to think, feel and act in certain ways,—that apart from any training the mind of its own accord or, to use a more technical word, instinctively behaves in certain ways under certain conditions.

For very many of the mind's connections we need no other immediate explanation than that human beings are by nature so organized as to manifest under certain cir-

[1] By some writers it is called *functional* psychology.

cumstances certain thoughts, feelings and acts. Just as human beings by nature possess arms and hands, so they possess nervous systems that lead them to reach for objects that lie within their view and to grasp the objects touched. Just as they are given by nature lips and tongues, so also they are given the feelings of sweetness and of pleasure thereat. Just as infants are given by nature muscles that turn the head and eyes, so they are given by nature a connection between seeing a light and turning the head and eyes toward it.

The capacity for becoming a great musician or a great orator or a great mathematician is to a large extent born in a man as a part of his original make-up. For all of the powers of sense, intellect and character there are certainly foundations in human nature apart from the training which life gives. Such features of our original make-up are due to the same causes as unlearned reactions.

The basis of a mind's action,—the starting point of the life of intellect, feeling and conduct,—is thus its equipment of instincts and capacities, its native or unlearned tendencies.

These correspond to qualities inherent in the nervous system, to characteristics of and connections between the neurones which are provided by nature. The brain is so constructed at birth and so grows by the inner impulse of development as to make stimulation of the neurones ending in the retina of the eye arouse sensations of light and color, to make the afferent nerve cells stimulated by the sight of a light connect with the motor cells that cause movements of the head and eyes toward the light. That we have, apart from training, a vast number of tendencies to feel and to act in certain ways in response to certain situations, corresponds to the fact that by the inner impulse of growth the brain is so made as to connect certain afferent neurones with certain associative and efferent neurones. That we have, apart from training, an equipment of capacities or possibilities of thought and action, corresponds to the fact that the brain is by nature fitted to do certain work.

Although much of human life finds its explanation in unlearned tendencies,—in the mental constitution provided by nature,—still more must be attributed to learning, experience, training. What is born in us soon becomes outweighed by what happens to us. The brain, the basis of mental life, is primarily an organ to be modified; the connections between its neurones are constantly being added to and substracted from; it is literally never the same at any two moments of life. The mind similarly is constantly adding and losing habits, increasing this and decreasing that capacity, changing with every influence that plays upon it. If we ask how the baby comes to feel pleasure at the sight of its mother, why we shut our eyes when told to do so or why we feel $30.00 to be more than 30 cents, the answer must be sought in the facts of the modification of connections by experience,—in the laws of mental acquisition.

The two great divisions of dynamic psychology will thus treat of: (1) The power of nature, manifested in instincts and capacities. (2) The power of nurture, manifested in habits and acquired powers.

CHAPTER XII

Original Tendencies to Connections

§ 31. *Instincts*

The Law of Instinct.—Instincts have been defined as all connections or tendencies to connections which are unlearned,—are in us apart from training or experience. The inborn constitution of a human being provides connections between certain situations and the responses made to them. The line of least resistance in any case will then, apart from training, be toward that response connected by nature with the situation. This fact may be called the *law of instinct* or the *law of original connections.* It may be stated as follows: In any situation that mental state or act will, other things being equal, take place which is by original nature most closely connected with the situation; or, the likelihood that any mental state or act will occur is, other things being equal, proportional to the closeness of its instinctive connection with the situation in question.

The Attributes of Instincts.—That an instinctive tendency is born in a human being as a result of the structure of his nervous system need not mean that it is present at birth. Creeping, standing erect and laughing are surely instinctive, but appear only after months of life. The new feelings and desires which characterize the change from childhood to adult life in the years from thirteen to sixteen are as truly instinctive as the infant's fears. The date of appearance of each instinct is a separate problem.

It is also an error to suppose that instinctive acts or feelings always jump suddenly into being, that what we do not learn we get in a flash as an instantaneous inspiration from nature. On the contrary, the common fact is a gradual growth. So, for instance, with the fear of strangers in young infants or the tendency to personal display with boys from fourteen to eighteen. There are all degrees of gradualness in the maturing of instincts.

Again, that a tendency is due to inborn nervous make-up need not mean that it will remain all through life. On the contrary, all instincts tend to die out if not given exercise, and may be killed off,—or, to use the technical term, inhibited,—when circumstances are so arranged that their manifestation leads to discomfort. Thus chicks brought up in isolation from the parent hen do not show, after ten or twelve days, the tendency to follow her; and children are taught by punishment to abandon their original tendency to grab every new and attractive object which they see. If an instinct does not accord with our notions of desirable behavior, we may and do get rid of it. If it is advantageous, we must take pains to provide the conditions to call it into use and to allow its action to result in pleasure. Instincts are a fund of capital loaned to us by nature for a period, not given outright. Only on the condition that they are used and bring satisfaction do they become our permanent property.

They become our permanent property by being hardened into habits. It is a general law of mind that any act or thought or feeling which in a given set of circumstances results in satisfaction, comfort or at least indifferently, is, if those circumstances recur, more likely to appear than in the first instance; and so on increasingly with more repetitions. The transitory instinct thus may become a permanent habit. The child who instinctively says *baba* or *mama* in its mother's presence and is rewarded by parental attention and petting, forms the habit of calling her by that name. The chick, in the ordinary course of events, follows the hen for a few days because of instinct, but from the second time on the force of habit combines with that of inner nature; so that by the eighth or tenth day, when the instinct, if left to itself, would have vanished, the chick continues the now habitual act.

It is common in books of natural history to give, as illustrations of instincts, extreme cases,—such as the building of the honeycomb by bees or the spinning of the web of the spider,—where the action is definite and uniform and highly specialized. But the majority of instincts are vague, variable and rough-hewn. The chick instinctively feeds itself by pecking at, picking up and swallowing small objects; but so far as the instinct goes, all sorts of small objects fit and unfit,—tacks, yarn, and match heads as well as seeds and bugs,—are pecked at. Experience, not instinct, decides the particular feeding-habits into which the vague instinct shall eventually grow.

This indefiniteness and lack of precise adaptation to any one particular situation is important because it allows the instinctive tendency to produce, not some one single habitual act, a replica of itself, but a number of different habits, each fitted to some special set of situations. Thus the vague, instinctive tendency of kittens when confined in boxes to squeeze, claw, bite and pull, gave rise to the habits of pulling a loop in one box, turning a button in another, pulling a lever in another, etc. Thus the general instinctive tendency of babies to take and pull and twist and turn and drop and poke all things grows into the multitude of habits of using toys and common household objects.

Akin to the naturalist's error of neglecting vague and variable instincts is the psychologist's error of neglecting general tendencies. The tendency of children to do all sorts of things to objects,—*e. g.*, to pull, turn, drop, pick up, roll, put in the mouth, bite, pull out and rub a new toy, —is as truly due to inborn make-up as are their tendencies to sneeze, laugh or creep. The instincts of the most importance to mental growth and education are those general tendencies to react in certain ways to large classes of experiences which we call curiosity, emulation and physical play.

Instincts, then, may be *delayed, gradual in appearing,* and *transitory;* they are *modifiable,* hardening into habits or becoming abolished by disuse or inhibition; they are often *indefinite* and *general.*

Human Instincts.—Too little is known about the extent to which human behavior is based upon instincts to allow their enumeration. But even with our present lack of knowledge the list of demonstrated instincts is a long one. It takes Professor James thirty-seven pages to list and describe them. Probably the list will grow with further study, since many actions which common sense credits to acquisition are really the gift of nature. *E. g.,* standing alone, walking and retrieving (getting an object and bringing it back) appear in babies who are given no incitement or assistance. The manifestations of grief,—puckering the lips, drawing down the face and a prolonged wail,—appear in babies at the stimulus of harsh speech or ugly looks, although such speech or looks have never been followed by any unpleasant consequence. The more carefully mental development is investigated, the more we find human life everywhere rooted in instincts.

Especially noteworthy in human instinctive equipment is the tendency which I shall call *multiple reaction to a single stimulus.* The reason for this name will appear from the following illustrations: The baby confronted by a small novel object, not only reaches and takes it; he also, as has already been noted, puts it in his mouth, takes it out, turns it over, drops it, picks it up, rolls it around, rubs it against his nose, looks at it in one way, then in another, holds it up, holds it down, and so on. Again the baby makes not a few distinct cries as does the dog or cat, but a rich variety of prattle, containing all sorts of combinations of sounds. By means of these multiple reactions to single stimuli the field of experimentation with things is far greater in man than in any other animal. Man, who does so many things to so many things, has the opportunity to develop a far wider range of habits. Out of the fumbling and prattle of the baby grow the play and speech of the child, and later the work and invention and thought of the man.

§ 32. *Capacities*

The Attributes of Capacities.—All the characteristics of instincts summarized in § 31 belong to the subtler possibilities of mental life which are called capacities. For instance, the capacity for managing men is delayed in comparison with that for acting or literary production. Apparently the capacity for seeing blue develops later than that for seeing other colors. Capacities of motor control and of sense perception have been proved to mature gradually. It is a common and likely belief that the capacity for rote-memorizing is transitory, weakening somewhat in spite of the tremendous amount of training which it receives. The capacity to adopt new points of view seems to be very often lost by the age of twenty-five. When their exercise is attended by pleasant results, capacities harden into actual powers, just as instincts harden into habits. The child with musical capacity, wisely trained, thus becomes capable of actual achievement in music. But disuse will as surely destroy the capacity, and the fact of a capacity positively stamped out by unpleasant results is one of the commonest facts in human life. Many men would have been great generals had there been wars enough. Most men could have been first-rate bullies and vagabonds, most women could have been first-rate coquettes, had not the capacities been stifled from childhood

It is fortunately true that useful capacities are not likely to be inhibited even when home and school offer them little encouragement. For the capacity itself begets interest, and mere achievement is often its sufficient reward. Sooner or later the boy or girl who has a capacity which the world needs will probably transform it into actual power and achievement. It is risky to console oneself for lack of success by the claim that one had as much capacity as anyone else but was not encouraged. There are, however, some sad cases of noble capacities starved and beaten to death.

The Specialization of Capacities.—Like instincts, capacities are often indefinite and generalized. Men are not born with the capacity to learn English or German, but to learn a language. Common belief, and many psychologists, however, make here an error just the reverse of that made concerning the same feature of instincts. In the latter case they overestimate the definiteness and specialization of inborn nature; in the case of capacities they overestimate the indefiniteness and generalization. These instincts of possibility are much more specialized than we commonly think or than the older books on psychology acknowledge. One may have the capacity to appreciate music without the capacity to appreciate other forms of art; one may be a most expert calculator with numerical problems and nearly an idiot in other fields of knowledge; a most gifted reasoner in mathematics was easily deceived by a spiritualist's tricks; the hardest-headed men of business are often silly in their superstitions; a most gifted and inventive scholar may be hopelessly stupid about the simplest bit of machinery.

§ 33. *Further Attributes of Original Tendencies*

Individual Differences in Inborn Nature.—Nature does not provide each human being with the same capital of instincts and capacities. Men are no more created alike in their mental constitutions than they are treated alike by their surroundings. Any instinct is possessed by different individuals in different degrees of strength. One is gentle, one harsh, one cruel, one a Nero. One strikes back only when teased for an hour, another at the least offense. Indeed there is probably no instinct which is not entirely lacking in some individuals. Even that one which is the first necessity for living, the suckling instinct, does not always appear. So also any capacity is possessed by different individuals in different degrees of strength, the variation here being even greater than in the case of instincts. Some men are born to be intellectual giants, some to be idiots. This is universally recognized only in such obvious cases as the capacities for music and poetry, but it is equally true of the capacity to add or to multiply, to read or to spell, to succeed in science or in affairs. Wherever measurements have been made of mental capacities, individual differences are the rule. In the keenness of the senses, in the quickness and accuracy of perception, in the vividness of imagery, in the permanence of memories, in the appreciation of relations,—everywhere men are by nature different. It is true that when thought of in comparison with other animals, men seem closely alike,—that amongst all men there is a general family resemblance. The differences amongst men seem small in comparison with the much greater difference between men and animals. But they exist, and in sufficient amount to explain a great part of the differences in human achievements.

The original mental equipment of any human individual is thus to be regarded as the result of two factors; (1) a fund of instincts and capacities which he has in common with other members of the human species, and which belongs to him as one of that species, and (2) an additional fund which belongs to him alone as an individual. It is most convenient to regard as the common fund, that which the ordinary, average, common man possesses and to regard any individual's special share as being either plus or minus. The common fund is then, not that possessed by all, but that possessed by the general type of the species. From this type an individual may deviate in either direction.

The Source of Original Nature.—So far the inborn equipment of instincts and capacities has been attributed to the constitution of the nervous system as determined by nature. We have now to ask what laws of nature control its distribution. These are *the law of heredity* and its supplement, *the law of variation.*

The mental constitution given by nature to any man is that of his ancestors plus many or few of the variations which occur in all living things. The special share characteristic of any individual,—his deviation from the general type of the species,—is his inheritance from his immediate ancestry; the common fund is his inheritance from his remote ancestry, the human race as a whole.

Much of this common fund dates its origin farther back than the human species. Just as the human backbone can be traced back to the notochord of Amphioxus, or the human kidney to the pronephros of the fishes, so many instincts and capacities can be traced back to our animal forebears. Scratching the head in perplexity is as old as the monkeys; creeping has a still more remote origin; the capacity to modify instincts into habits is an inheritance fully as old as the backbone. We are by nature a part of a species thousands of years old,—a part, too, of the animal kingdom as a whole. In mind as in body, man bears the marks of his long ascent.

The special characteristics of an individual are partly due to normal variation and partly to the characteristics of his immediate ancestors. The second factor is by far the greater. Measurements of the resemblance of parents to offspring and of brother to brother prove that, in the same way and for the same reason that tall parents have tall children or dark-haired parents dark-haired children, so also stupid parents have stupid children, hot-tempered parents have hot-tempered children, and musical parents, musical children.

Original mental make-up is thus determined by heredity, slightly supplemented by chance variation. To it prehuman species contribute; the thousands of generations of savage and prehistoric man add their shares; its special features in any individual are the bequests of his nearer ancestry. On this foundation of original make-up, nurture builds. The bequests of heredity are invested and made productive by the environment. Instincts and capacities are modified and transformed by experience. The study of the laws by which this modification takes place will occupy us in the next six chapters.

The Control of Original Tendencies.—Although instincts and capacities are, in and of themselves, removed from human control, their later modifications are not. They are a fund of capital given by nature which may be invested in all sorts of ways. We make the most of nature's gifts by (1) encouraging the useful instincts and capacities, (2) inhibiting the harmful ones, and (3) by so arranging life's work as to have natural tendencies assist rather than oppose it.

(1) Useful instincts and capacities are encouraged: (a) by being given exercise as soon as they appear and frequently enough to result in the formation of habits before the instinct wanes, and (b) by making their consequences pleasurable.

(2) Harmful instincts and capacities are weakened or inhibited: (a) by depriving them of exercise, by not allowing the situations which would evoke them to appear, (b) by forming, before the tendency is fixed, the habit of meeting the situation in some other way, and (c) by making their consequences intolerable.

(3) No general answer can be given to the question suggested by (3), but one or two illustrations will show the gain to be everywhere expected from recognition of and allowance for natural tendencies. A man wanted a pile of rocks removed. He taught his boys to play that there was a fire in a hole some distance away and that the rocks were pails of water and they the firemen. In a few days not a rock was left. At a city playground the older boys bullied and teased the younger ones. The sagacious director picked out several leaders from among the older boys and appointed them policemen to enforce fairness

and to protect the "little kids." The instincts of activity and combativeness and emulation were now turned to useful ends. Bullying the small boys gave way to governing the large ones. Judge Lindsey of Denver turns youthful offenders into arms of the law by directing the instinctive love of excitement into the channel of detective work against men selling liquor to minors.

The individual differences in inborn original nature may be prevented from waste and made to do service by specialization in the home, in school, in business—in fact everywhere. Since men are different, they are adapted to different careers in life. By finding out their individual constitutions and directing their energies in appropriate channels, we may make them happier and more useful, may preserve them from unmeaning instruction and profitless tasks and incite them to service which they can do better than anyone else.

Exercises

1. Pugnacity, climbing, walking, emulation, jealousy, biting the finger nails, curiosity, and manipulation or constructiveness are commonly quoted cases of instinctive tendencies. What are the situations and the responses, the connections of which constitute these several instincts? *E. g.*, pugnacity means the response, 'blow,' to the situation, 'being injured or interfered with,' and the response, 'enjoyment,' to the situation, 'fighting.'

2. Of the instincts named in question 1, name one that is delayed, one that is transitory, one that is common to man and the lower animals, one that is specially characteristic of the male sex, one that is most useful, one that is often the origin of criminal acts.

3. Give two illustrations from history or from your own acquaintance of a high degree of capacity coupled with only moderate attainments in other directions.

4. Just how would you get rid of the tendency in a child to torment animals? After writing your answer read again (2) of

page 196 and note which methods of those mentioned there your plan involves.

5. Which is rarer, the capacity to form percepts or the capacity to form abstract ideas?

6. Illustrate individual differences (a) in the case of sensation, and (b) in the case of imagery.

7. Illustrate race heredity, *i. e.,* the inheritance of certain mental qualities by a race as a whole.

Experiment 17. Instincts of the Reflex Type.—Have a friend hold about half or three quarters of an inch in front of his eyes, a piece of glass, at least an eighth of an inch thick. Throw directly at his eye a bit of cork or light wood, or a small wad of paper, so aimed that, but for the glass, it would hit the eye and at a fair rate of speed. Of course he winks.

Then inform him that you will repeat the process, and that since it is impossible that anything can hit his eye he is to keep it wide open. Throw as before. Is the eye kept open? Repeat nine times more, noting and recording each time the action of the eyelids.

Experiment 18. The Modifiability of Instincts.—With sufficient time the instinctive closing of the eye can be modified and even inhibited. The experiment may take many trials. If it is made, a tube like a pea-shooter, but one half inch in diameter and not over eight inches long, and a sufficient number of bits of cork about a quarter of an inch in diameter, should be provided.

Record the action of the eyelids at each trial, and continue the experiment until the person can hold the eyelids unmoved during ten successive trials.

References

A. James, *Briefer Course,* XXV.
Titchener, *Outline,* §§ 35, 66-67.
Angell, *Psychology,* XV., XVI.
B. James, *Principles,* XXIV.

CHAPTER XIII

The Law of Association

§ 34. *The Growth of Instincts into Habits*

Under the influence of the outside conditions that form human nature, instincts and capacities grow into an almost countless multitude of habits of thought, feeling and action. On the basis of our many unlearned tendencies, we learn still more numerous acts and ideas. To original equipment is added the store of knowledge and skill which we acquire. How this modification and development of instincts and capacities into the fullness of mental life is brought to pass is the subject of this chapter.

Some Concrete Cases.—A simple case of the development of habits from instincts will introduce us best to the laws that govern this process. A child eight months old was kept an hour or so each day in a chair beside a window. To a cord hung from above were attached some of his playthings. His instinctive tendency led him to pull at, poke and finger these. By a specially vigorous pull to one side the toy would be swung against the window glass. This sort of a pull occurred occasionally among the many acts which resulted from his instinctive play. It noticeably attracted the child's attention and aroused the expression of satisfaction. As time went on he did it oftener and oftener until swinging the toy against the glass became a regular feature of his play. The vague instinctive pulling had given birth to a special habit.

The particular act of pulling in a certain way had been selected from the many acts performed and had been associated more and more closely with the situation 'being in that chair in sight of that string of toys.' The force which strengthened the connection between that particular act and the situation was not only its repetition, but also the resultant satisfaction, for other acts done as frequently at the beginning faded out and did not result in any new habits. This will be still clearer from two illustrations drawn from animal life.

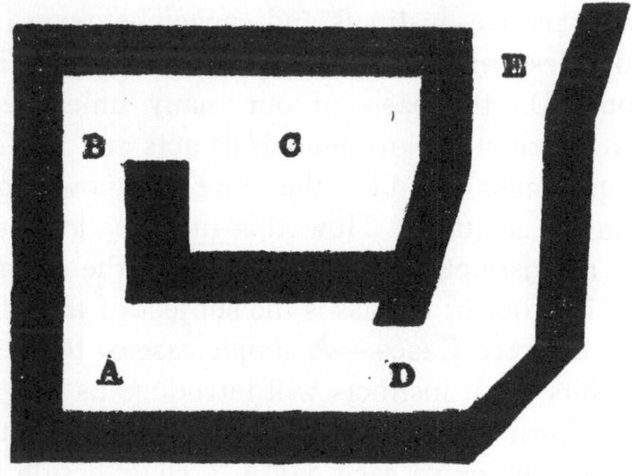

FIG. 74.

"If we make a pen, as shown in Fig. 74, and put but a chick, say six days old, in at *A,* it is confronted by a situation which is, briefly, 'the sense-impression or feeling of the confining surfaces, an uncomfortable feeling due to the absence of other chicks and of food, and perhaps the sense-impressions of the chirping of the chicks outside.' It reacts in this situation by running around, making loud sounds, and jumping at the walls. When it jumps at the walls, it has uncomfortable feelings of effort; when it runs to *B,* or *C,* or *D,* it has a continuation of the feelings of the situation just described; when it runs to *E,* it gets out, feels the pleasure of being with the other chicks, of the taste of food, of being in its usual habitat. If from time to time you put it in again, you find that it jumps and runs to *B, C,* and *D* less and less often, until finally its only act is to run to *D, E,* and out. It has, to use technical psychological terms, formed an association between the sense-impression or situation due to its presence at *A* and the act of going to *E*. In common language it has *learned* to go to *E* when put at *A*—has learned the way out. The decrease in the useless runnings and jumping and standing still finds a representative in the decreasing amount of time taken by the chick to escape. The two chicks that formed this particular association, for example, averaged one about three and the other about four minutes for their first five trials, but came finally to escape invariably within five or six seconds.

The following schemes represent the animal's behavior (1) during an early trial and (2) after the association has been fully formed—after it has learned perfectly the way out.

(1)

SITUATION	IMPULSES	ACTS	RESULTING FEELINGS
As described above.	To chirp, etc. To jump at various places. To run to *B*. " " " *C*. " " " *D*.	Corresponding to impulses.	Continuation of situation. Fatigue.
	" " " *E*.		Pleasure of company. " " food. " " surroundings.

(2)

SITUATION	IMPULSES	ACTS	RESULTING FEELINGS
Same as (1).	To run to *E*.	Corresponding to impulse.	Pleasurable as above.

If we take a box twenty by fifteen by twelve inches, replace its cover and front side by bars an inch apart, and make in this front side a door arranged so as to fall open when a wooden button inside is turned from a vertical to a horizontal position, we shall have means to observe another simple case of learning. A kitten, three to six months old, if put in this box when hungry, a bit of fish being left outside, reacts as follows: It tries to squeeze through between the bars, claws at the bars and at loose things in and out of the box, reaches its paws out between the bars, and bites at its confining walls. Some one of all these promiscuous clawings, squeezings, and bitings turns round the wooden button, and the kitten gains freedom and food. By repeating the experience again and again, the animal gradually comes to omit all the useless clawings, etc., and to manifest only the particular impulse (*e. g.*, to claw hard at the top of the button with the paw, or to push against one side of it with the nose) which has resulted successfully. It turns the button round without delay whenever put in the box. It has formed an association between the situation, 'confinement in a box of a certain appearance,' and the impulse to the act of clawing at a certain part of that box in a certain definite way. Popularly speaking, it has learned to open a door by turning a button. To the uninitiated observer the behavior of the six kittens that thus freed themselves from such a box would seem wonderful and quite unlike their ordinary accomplishments of finding their way to their food, beds, etc., but the reader will realize that the activity is of just the same sort as that displayed by the chick in the pen. A certain situation arouses, by virtue of accident, or, more often, instinctive equipment certain impulses and corresponding acts. One of these happens to be an act appropriate to secure freedom. It is stamped in in connection with that situation. Here the act is 'clawing at a certain spot' instead of 'running to *E*,' and is selected from a far greater number of useless acts."[1]

The Law of Habit-Formation.—The characteristics of these cases of learning are that from the instinctive tendencies present the one which brings satisfaction is selected and is associated more and more closely with the situation until it alone is the reaction to that situation. The tendencies which bring discomfort are more and more dissociated from that situation until they may be totally eliminated and never appear in response to it. *Selection* and *Association* best describe the process. *Satisfaction* best describes the motive force in it. The result is that a set of special habits or connections between each particular situation and its fitting response takes the place of the original vague instinct.

Instincts are thus modified into habits in accordance with the law that *any act which in a given situation produces satisfaction becomes associated with that situation, so that when the situation recurs the act is more likely than before to recur also.* Conversely, *any act which in a given situation produces discomfort becomes dissociated from that situation, so that when the situation recurs the act is less likely than before to recur.*

The case is the same when the response to the situation is a thought or feeling instead of an act. So the law may be stated, *any mental state or act* which, etc.

§ 35. *The Formation of Connections in General*

Habits Formed From Previous Habits.—The same process of learning occurs when the development is not from mere instinctive tendencies but from these as modified by previous training. The baby who has formed the

[1] E. L. Thorndike in the *Woods Holl Biological Lectures for 1899*, pp. 70-74.

habit of swinging a toy against the window-pane may later, as an outgrowth of that habit, form the new habit of swinging the toy rhythmically. The process is again simply the selection of the rhythmical movement from amongst the many sorts made because of its relatively greater amount of resulting satisfaction. We may therefore widen the statement of our law and say:—In any situation the thoughts, feelings and acts manifested will be those to which instinctive tendencies or capacities *and also previously formed habits* impel one. Of all these the one which succeeds best, results in the most satisfaction, will be associated with that situation.

Some Additions to the Law of Habit Formation.—In some cases the results of original tendencies and previous learning will be to furnish, not a number of acts,—some more, some less, some not at all fitted to the situation,—but to arouse directly the one suitable act. For instance, the chicken a few days old in the presence of a worm does not pick at it in many different ways, some quite useless; he at once seizes it. The baby may suckle at once when the breast is offered to it. In such cases the selection is of one act from one only. The formation of the habit means as before the strengthening of one connection, though not the exclusion of other connections.

Resulting satisfaction is not always a *sine qua non* in the formation of connections. Mere repetition strengthens the connection between situation and response, provided no positive discomfort results. The child who says dog at the sight of the letters d o g often enough, will learn to do so even though he has never obtained any observable benefit from so doing. The law then may be stated, 'which in a given situation *does not produce discomfort.*' The greater the satisfaction produced, however, the more firmly will the connection be made between the response and its situation, and vice versa. Thus amended the law becomes:—Any mental state or act which in a given situation does not produce discomfort becomes associated with that situation, so that when the situation recurs the mental state or act is more likely than before to recur also; the greater the satisfaction produced by it, the stronger the association. Conversely, any mental state or act which in a given situation does produce discomfort becomes disconnected from that situation, so that when the situation recurs the mental state or act is less likely than before to recur also; the greater the discomfort produced by it, the weaker the association becomes.

From another point of view the law may be stated as: *In any situation the mental state or act will take place which has resulted from that situation oftenest and with the most satisfaction.*

The law of habit formation and the law of instinctive connection may be combined into one as follows: *The likelihood that any mental state or act will occur in response to any situation is in proportion to the closeness of its inborn connection therewith, to the frequency of its connection therewith, and to the amount of satisfaction resulting.* This may be called the *Law of Least Resistance in Mental Life.*

The Real Situation May Be More or Less Than the Apparent Situation.—The word situation in the law of instinct and the law of association must be taken broadly. The connection made is not necessarily with one particular circumstance or thing, but often is with the total state of affairs felt. Thus the chicken in the pen whose behavior was described in § 34, did not make connection with the situation, 'sight of confining walls,' but rather with the situation, sight of confining walls plus feelings of hunger plus absence of sight of companions plus sound of companions at a distance plus absence of food.' The same particular circumstance may in one set of surrounding circumstances,—in one mental context,—connect with one act and in a different mental context, with another. Had the chick been put into a pen with other chicks and food, it would have played about and pecked at the food and only occasionally jumped at the confining walls. The sight of the figures below (Fig. 75) would call up in a school-boy's mind the thoughts of a cube and a sphere if felt in connection with the surroundings of his school room and geometry class, while if felt in connection with the ordinary sights of street or playroom they would call up the thought of a box and a ball.

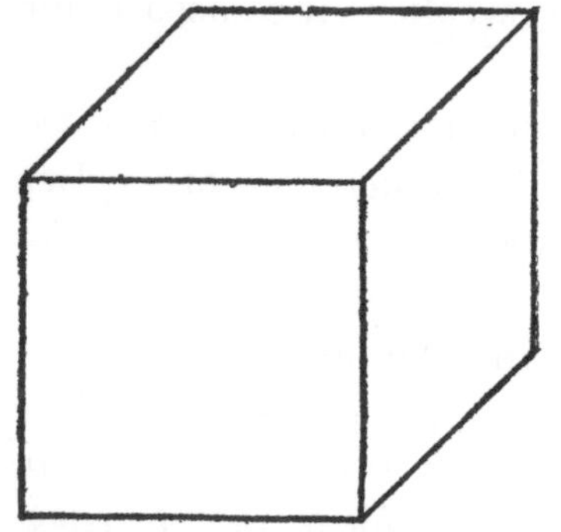

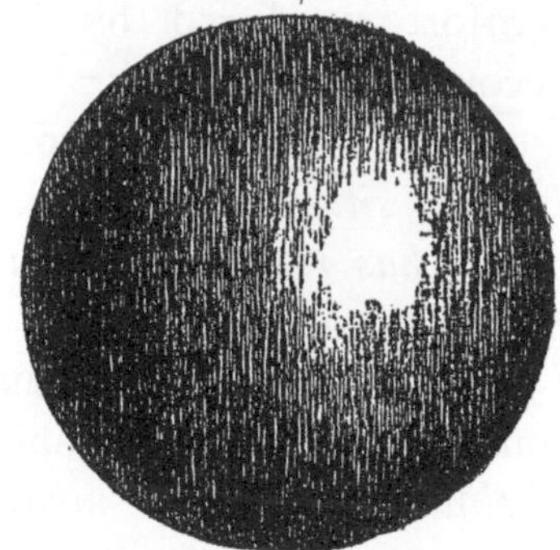

Fig. 75.

The situation may then be the whole state of mind, the circumstances or thing in its context, the entire 'attitude' or 'set' of mental life, as well as the particular fact in its focus.

On the other hand the connection made may be with some very small element of the apparent situation. In learning to swim the connections are not made with the color, temperature, taste and smell of the water, but only with the feelings of non-solidity, of suspension and of sinking. In learning to play a piece on the piano the connections are not made with the color of the instrument, the quality of the room's atmosphere and the size of the music book, but with the position of the notes on the scale, the form of the notes, the feelings of one's arms and fingers and the sounds produced.

The facts that the connection may be made not only with the apparent situation, but also with it plus the co-operating attitude of the mind as a whole or with it minus many or all but one of its elements may be stated as the laws (1) *of the Mind's Set* and (2) *of Partial Activity*. These are:—

(1) *The likelihood that any mental state or act will occur in response to any apparent situation is in proportion to the closeness of its connection with the total set of the mind at the time as well as with the apparent situation itself.*

(2) *The likelihood that any mental state or act will occur in response to any apparent situation is in proportion to the closeness of its connection with the apparent situation or some element or part thereof.*

Recency and Intensity of Connections.—Other factors besides the results of a connection and its frequency determine the likelihood of its operation, namely, recency and intensity. For the sake of simplicity these factors may remain undescribed until later chapters. An adequate statement of the entire *Law of Association* would be: THE LIKELIHOOD THAT ANY MENTAL STATE OR ACT WILL OCCUR IN RESPONSE TO ANY SITUATION IS IN PROPORTION TO THE FREQUENCY, RECENCY, INTENSITY AND RESULTING SATISFACTION OF ITS CONNECTION WITH THAT SITUATION OR SOME PART OF IT AND WITH THE TOTAL FRAME OF MIND IN WHICH THE SITUATION IS FELT.

The Varieties of Connections.—The law of association applies not only to the growth of connections between sensory situations and responses to them, but also to the growth of all the forms of connections described in Chapter I.

Connections between (1) physical stimuli and mental states, between (2) one mental state and another, between (3) ideas and acts—all are formed in accordance with the law of association. Illustrations of (1) need some preliminary explanation and will be reserved for another chapter (Chapter XV). Illustrations of (2) are found in almost every process of memory or thought. We think of 36 when we think of 9×4 because with the situation, 'thinking of 9×4' the thought of 36 has gone oftenest and with most satisfaction. Illustrations of (3) are found in almost every hour of daily life. We start for the class-room when the clock strikes the hour because we have done so; when we feel a desire to read, we buy a magazine because we have done so and with pleasurable results.

In cases where the connection involves a bodily act, it will be found that the satisfaction or discomfort resulting plays a large part in the formation or breaking of the connection. In cases where the connection involves only thoughts and feelings, the mere frequency of the response will be found to play the leading rôle. This is due to the fact that (1) the satisfaction resulting from responding to a situation by a successful idea so often comes much later. The boy in school who thinks of the correct answer to a question does not feel much satisfaction at the time. Often he does not know that his idea is right and so feels none. It is later when he is asked to recite and wins approval, or when his examination paper is returned and he finds it marked high, that the satisfaction comes. Moreover (2) the results of many of our mental responses produce almost no satisfaction. It makes little difference whether the sight of a watch arouses the thought of a clock or the thought of time or the thought of wheels; whether the thought of John arouses the thought of Smith or of Jones or of Anderson.

§ 36. *The Control of the Formation of Connections*

Three Essentials in Efficient Learning.—The applications of the law of association to the control of mental life by school education and general training are clear. In briefest terms they are as follows:—

The first necessity of mental progress is fertility in response. Unless the baby does something, it can learn nothing; there is nothing for selection to work upon. Intellect and character cannot be created from a void. Other things being equal, the capacity for varied responses, great activity, curiosity, and mental energy increase the probability of mental improvement.

The second means of training is the arrangement of instructive situations,—of conditions the responses to which may form valuable associations. As civilization progresses, men try increasingly to provide in the home, in schools and in the world's affairs, situations fitted to induce profitable responses. The behavior and conversation of the people about us, the books, laboratories, museums and other school paraphernalia, sermons, newspapers, music, laws and the like—all aim to control the mind's acts by controlling the situations to which it responds. In the words of a sagacious trainer of animals, we "Arrange all the circumstances of the experiment so that the animal is compelled by the laws of its own nature to do the trick."

The third means is the arrangement of the results of

the different possible responses so that desirable ones give satisfaction and undesirable ones, discomfort. By rewards and punishments, natural or designed, parents, teachers, employers and rulers preserve the responses which they approve and stamp out those which they disapprove. The history of a mind's training is in great measure the history of the elimination of its mistakes.

These Three Factors Illustrated.—These three factors may be illustrated by almost any mental achievement, for instance, by learning to read. The teacher arranges a chart with a picture of a cat, the word cat and the like. The more skillfully she can arrange to get the situation 'attention to the picture, the c a t and the sound as she or some pupil pronounces it,' the better the prospect that the associations between the c a t and the picture and sound will be formed. If now there is an utterly stolid, idiotic boy who is aroused to no action by the situation, who does not look at the chart or listen to the teacher, or repeat the sound after her, or think of cats or dogs or anything else, the process of teaching him to read is blocked at the outset and cannot progress till he is somehow stimulated to respond.

Usually, of course, responses will be made; the children will say *cat* when the picture is pointed out, will repeat *cat* after the teacher when she points at the word and says *cat;* and will say *cat* when she points at the word but says nothing; some may however say 'kitten,' or 'What is that?' or the last word the teacher has herself said. If the teacher looked as pleased, and said yes as often, and in general rewarded these incorrect replies as she does the correct ones, the process would again be blocked. It is the satisfaction or discomfort which she causes that selects the sound *cat* to be the permanent fixed associate of the sight c a t.

§ 37. *Response by Analogy*

Responses to Novel Situations.—The law of instinct and the law of association fail apparently to prophesy what will happen when a situation appears for which no instinctive connection exists and which has never before been experienced. What, for example, will a chicken do when it for the first time sees a piece of yarn? What will a student unlearned in zoölogy do who is asked to name the picture of an Amphioxus?

There being no response provided for that particular situation by inborn constitution[1] or previous experience, the individual *will respond as he would to some situation like it,* to which instinct or training has provided a response. The chicken will respond to the yarn as he would instinctively to a worm, will seize it, run away and begin to swallow it. The student will call the picture of Amphioxus a worm, though it is not, because experience has connected the word worm with long, legless, finless things.

Every stimulus tends to discharge in some response; and in default of any response specially connected with it by nature or nurture, a stimulus will discharge into that response which has gone with something like it. This fact, that any unprepared-for situation will be treated as some familiar one like it would be, may be called *Assimilation* or *Response by Analogy.* The fact may be stated more exactly as follows:—

To any situation for which neither nature nor nurture provides a response the response will be that which they provide for the situation most like it; or, *Any situation*

[1] It must be remembered that for many new situations there is provided an instinctive response just because of their novelty. 'To handle and look at' is the baby's instinctive reaction to small novel objects as a class.

which has by nature and nurture no connections will connect with that response which the situation most like it would connect with.

Response by Analogy.—Learning to deal with new situations is a constant repetition of the following process: the new is treated as some situation like it would be treated; by the results of the responses the responses themselves are modified until in due time a response is selected that is well adapted to the situation.

The probable physiological basis for assimilation is easy to conceive, though proof is absent. Let us call the stimulation set up in the neurones by the new situation A B C D E F G. For just this particular situation there is no response provided; with just this neurone-group action there is no connection formed. But suppose that for the brain action A K C D E F G, there is a connection formed, M N O. The line of least resistance, of strongest connection for A B C D E F G would be toward M N O rather than toward some other; for the elements A C D E F and G would tend each to call up its own connection. The fact that the new situation resembles some other means that it has elements in common with some other. It can call up a response because these elements *do* have some formed connection though it as a whole has not. It calls up the response which would be made to the situation most like it, because being most like it means containing many of the elements which it contains. The elements in it call up the response which they are connected with, namely, the response made to the situation most like it. Assimilation, then, is one instance of the *law of partial activity.* The case may be likened roughly to that of the direction taken by a four horse team at a fork in the roads, when the team has never traveled either road *as a team* but some one horse or a pair *has.* Their previous habit of taking, say, the left turn, will cause the whole team to go that way.

The law of response by analogy is of importance apart from its service as an account of the means of responses to new situations; for even when instinct or habit does furnish a response, that response may be neglected in favor of the response which would be made to some situation resembling the one present. The baby who on seeing a bottle of small white medicine-tablets sang out 'shirt buttons' could have followed instinct and responded merely by fumbling and biting the new things. The school boy who, when asked to give the opposite of frequently, wrote 'a bad smell,' could have followed previous habits and said, 'I don't know.'

Exercises

1. What addition should be made to the maxim, "Practice makes perfect?"

2. Why is repetition more useful in acquiring knowledge than in acquiring skill?

3. Show how the law of association applies (a) to learning to ride a bicycle, (b) to learning to be tactful in dealing with people, (c) to learning to read, (d) to learning to shoot straight.

4. (a) Give two cases of learning in which resultant satisfaction is the main factor. (b) Give two cases in which resulting discomfort is the main factor. (c) Give two cases in which frequency is the main factor.

5. Give two illustrations of the law of the mind's set. Give two illustrations of the law of partial activity.

6. Explain by the laws described in this chapter or the preceding one the following facts:

a. The existence of the so-called 'happy families'; *e. g.*, of dogs, cats, mice, chickens, living together in peace.

b. That a religion based on fear commonly produces only negative morality; *i. e.*, only the absence of evil, not the presence of good acts.

c. Young children (five to eight years old) will commonly

define an object by its use. Thus a knife 'is a thing to cut with', a chair 'is what you sit on'.

d. A child in the primary class of a school committed some misdemeanor and was called to the teacher's desk and punished. A day or so later when occasion offered he committed the same fault but when told to come to the teacher's desk sat stubbornly still.

e. A child from the country who was being shown the animals in the zoological gardens called the antelopes calves.

7. In what way does attention play a part in acquisitions by the law of association?

8. Criticise the following statement:

"Our nervous system grows to the modes in which it has been exercised."

9. The probable physical parallel in the nervous system for the law of association is the law of the formation of connections stated and described in Chapter X. Read again § 27 and for each feature of the law of association find the probable physiological parallel.

References

A. James, *Briefer Course,* X.
Stout, *Manual,* 76-96.
B. James, *Principles,* IV.

CHAPTER XIV

The Law of Dissociation or Analysis

§ 38. *The Process of Analysis*

Important as is the action of the mind in connecting impressions with ideas and acts, ideas with ideas and acts and acts among themselves, it would be a gross mistake to restrict mental action to the single field of connections, habit formation, association. The mind works not only by association, by connecting this situation with that response, but also by *dis*sociation or analysis, by breaking up a total situation into its elements. The abstract and general notions which we found in Part I to be essential features in the higher types of human thinking and the operations of parts of impressions or ideas which will later be found to be essential features of reasoning, are mental products which come, not by putting things together, but by separating them into parts. The bare facts of experience give only white paper, white balls, white liquids, never the thought of mere whiteness by itself; the law of association, so far as hitherto described, would lead to an interminable repetition of selections from our experience and responses, never to the original insights of the mathematical or scientific thinker; the same law in conduct would provide only a better and better selection from amongst acts, a greater skill due to the elimination of failures, never with totally new moral insights or new combinations of bodily movements. But in fact we do separate out elements in thought which have never appeared before by themselves, but only as parts or elements of total experiences. We do come to make isolated movements which have previously been only parts of instinctive and habitual reactions. And this work of analysis of total impressions into ideas of parts and elements and qualities and of complex acts into minute separate movements is of the utmost use in giving command over the problems of thought and the activities of the body. By dividing we conquer. How this process of analysis occurs will be clear from a few simple cases.

The child at school whom we wish to feel the abstract quality of sphericity is given marbles and balls to observe. His attention is called to the orange, the gas globe, and the like. The word round or sphere is associated with all these and other objects, alike in being spheres but different in size, color, use, etc. As a result he comes to feel in connection with the word the special quality of similarity of surface at all points which to him means sphericity. Again the child to whom we wish to teach the abstract thing, number,—for instance the abstract quality of fiveness,—is given five peas, five sticks, five leaves, is made to draw five lines, to move his arm five times, to hold up five fingers, each time in association with the word five. He comes, by having the five quality constantly present but in connection with all sorts of other accessory qualities, to feel the numerical aspect of any group, the five aspect, by itself as a separate elementary thought in his mind.

In movements the same procedure is followed. A backward child can say *th* in common words but cannot make by themselves the movements needed to produce it alone. He is led to repeat *that, those, they, this, then, breathe* and similar words in order to lift into separate existence the *th* movement, to develop direct control of it.

In all these cases the method taken to develop into a separate idea or act some aspect of a total mental state or muscular performance,—to abstract, that is, some part or quality of an experience,—is to arouse many experiences in which that aspect or part or quality is constantly present but with in each case different surroundings or context. The element of idea or impulse which is thus felt with many different associates comes to be felt with none of them, to be felt by itself as an idea, to be independent of any of them. The movement which is thus made with many different associated movements comes to be made by itself alone. B A C D, E A F G, H A I J, K A L M, etc., result in a new A.

It thus seems to be the general law of mind that *any element of mental life which is felt as a part of many total mental states, differing in all else save its presence, comes thereby to be felt as an idea by itself, and that any movement which has been made as a part of many complex movements differing in all else save its presence comes thereby to be made as a movement by itself.* This law is called the law of *Dissociation by Varying Concomitants,* or the *Law of Analysis.*[1]

§ 39. *The Influence of the Law of Analysis*

In the arithmetic of the primary school where the meanings of the numbers from one to twenty and their

[1] The law of dissociation is really only one case of the law of association; it is the multitude of connections which serves to disconnect. The same general principle accounts for both association and dissociation, although the results of its workings are opposite in the two cases. When one thing has gone with another it tends to call it up and to fuse with it; but when one thing has gone with many different others it will tend to call up each of them a little and so none of them fully, and, instead of fusing with any one of them, to win an independent existence.

combinations are taught; in all inductive work in science where a general law or general notion is evolved from particular series of events or cases; in learning the meaning of but, and, notwithstanding, in spite of, etc., from their use in conversation and books; in comparing one character in literature or history with others to bring out essential points of his make-up—in short in all cases where we try to progress from vague feelings of a total fact to exact, definite feelings of its elements and of it as the compound of those elements—we depend upon the law of analysis or dissociation.

This law is the basis of the capacity to reason, *i.e.*, to think out the solutions of novel problems. Indeed it is probable that to the workings of this law of dissociation in infancy is due the growth of thought itself and of all those mental states which we call ideas,—that but for it mental life would be entirely composed of feelings like dizziness, suffocation, nausea, weariness or faintness, feelings which we would be very conscious of and would react to violently, but which we could not turn into continued and useful thought.

The infant's feelings of things, qualities, conditions and relationships are nothing more than vague total impressions of this person, that thing, this weather, that stomach-ache and the like. Only after many experiences, resulting in many associations and comparisons, have given the law of dissociation an opportunity to play its rôle, does he come to feel the sense qualities of objects as discriminated elements, to feel forms and colors and sizes and shapes distinct from each other. His bottle, for instance, is to him for months only a vaguely sizable thing to be taken and held in his mouth. Only after much experience does it become a thing so long, so heavy and so colored. Even in adults much of mental life never develops into definite ideas. How few, for example, are the smells which we feel as definitely in the general odor of a cook shop as we do red and green in the colors of a landscape.

As the infant gradually dissociates the elements of color, form, size and the like from the complex things in which they inhere, so the school boy in long years dissociates the more abstract qualities, such as justice, law or liberty. And to the end of life a thinking man will be busy in analyzing his vague impressions and opinions into their elements.

The elements acquired by the action of the law of dissociation furnish new materials for the law of association to work with. As soon as the child in school feels the meanings of 1, 2, 3, 4 and 5, he is ready to form the associations 1 and 2 are 3, 1 and 3 are four, 1 and 4 are 5, 2 and 3 are 5. As soon as a new movement comes under control, *i.e.*, can be made by itself, it enters into associations with other movements and with mental states. The first mental connections are between particular sensory situations and responses thereto, simple modifications of existing instincts. Starting with these the law of dissociation produces the feelings of common objects, qualities, acts and relations, such as children commonly manifest in the third year of life. These new feelings as fast as they appear become associated with words, acts and with each other, so that the child by the time of entrance to school has thousands of associations between ideas, mostly between concrete particulars. With these associations further action of the law of dissociation produces general and abstract ideas. These in turn form new associations. Thus in mental growth connection and analysis, association and dissociation, putting things together and breaking things up into parts, constantly work together.

§ 40. *The Control of the Process of Analysis*

The conditions favoring the analysis of a definite element out of a vague and complex total fact are:—

1. The collection of a number of total facts in each of which (a) the element is as obtrusive as possible, as little encumbered by irrelevant detail as possible and in which (b) the element's concomitants or surroundings vary. Thus if the teacher wishes to develop in a pupil's mind the abstract idea of the passive voice, he uses such examples as: *he is struck, they were accepted, you will be applauded, Grant was elected,* rather than the repetition four times of, *I am satisfied.* For in the last example the passive element is not at all prominent; the pupil may well think of satisfied as an adjective; and the element is not thrown into relief by variations in the other features of the examples.

2. That these facts be compared with attention directed toward the parts or elements of each fact, especially toward the element in question. In the illustration above, attention could readily be directed toward the passive voice aspect by comparing the four sentences each with its corresponding active (he is struck, he strikes; they were accepted, they accepted, etc.)

3. That a symbol or name of some kind be ready to be associated with the element when felt. Unconnected feelings cannot maintain an existence in the mind; a fact thought of without a name of some sort is just an unconnected feeling. Let me have never so clear an idea of the thing, I shall gain by having also associated with it a name. So in the illustration above good teachers are

careful to give the name 'passive voice' as soon as the pupil has the feeling, 'subject does nothing, something is done to him.'

To assure the permanence of the feeling, repeated practice in detecting the element in new complexes is necessary. So the teacher sets the pupil to pick out all the passives he can on a page, or to divide a mixed list into actives and passives, or to perform some other exercise to the same end.

The conditions that favor analysis are thus those that would be met by a fertile and selective mind, one that would naturally summon together many facts and attend to their parts. More is required here than for the simple association of ideas and acts. Hence the capacity to dissociate or analyze is of later and higher development. Animals possessing the former lack it. Babies form many associative habits before they show any signs of analysis. In feeble minded adults analysis develops only to a slight extent. The commonest sense elements, such as color, size, shape, few, many, and the like, are known, but to feel the meaning of 'twenty,' or of 'a promise' or of 'opposite' is beyond their power. In individuals of high intellectual ability, on the other hand, the process of dissociation is very prominent.

Exercises

1. Which process, association or dissociation, is involved in each of the following?
   - (a) in learning to ride a bicycle.
   - (b) in learning a poem by heart.
   - (c) in learning to understand the difference between the present tense and the past tense.
   - (d) in learning to understand the difference between *by* to express means and *by* to express agency.
   - (e) in learning the meanings of the numbers.

(f) in learning the multiplication table.
(g) in learning the meanings of velocity and of acceleration.
(h) in learning to spell.

2. For which is dissociation more necessary, (a) learning the grammar of a language or learning its vocabulaory? (b) Learning algebra or learning geometry? (c) Learning physical geography or learning commercial geography?

3. (a) What associations would be necessary before a child could by dissociation come to feel the meaning of *if?* (b) Of *longer than?* (c) Of *positive, comparative* and *superlative?*

4. How would you develop in the mind of a school-boy a definite and independent idea of acceleration, or of wealth, or of reciprocity?

References

A. James, *Briefer Course,* XV.
B. James, *Principles,* XIII. (502-508).

§ 41. *Physiological Conditions of Human Nature*

The three laws presented in this and the two preceding chapters summarize the method of action of nature and nurture, inborn mental constitution and acquired modifications, in its most essential features. The intellect and character of any one of us is due largely to the operation of these three laws. Not entirely, however; for any human being's thought and conduct, depending as they do upon the action of his nervous system, will sometimes show mysterious alterations,—behavior unexplainable by the laws of instinct, association and dissociation. The nervous system is influenced not only by the factors accounted for in these three laws, but also by fatigue, drugs, sickness, the decay of old age, shock, the chance variations of blood-pressure, metabolism and the like.

It is necessary in a brief treatment to omit the facts that are known concerning the action of these forces, as well as the many problems answers to which are yet to be discovered. I have used and shall in the future, frequently use the phrase *'other things being equal'* to recall to the reader's mind the fact that there are always many complex possibilities for mental action at any moment. Even when no such provisional clause is in the text the reader should supply it mentally. He should not forget, for instance, that though the general law of mental life is the law of association or habit, a sufficient dose of hashish will keep in temporary abeyance the most fixed habits of perception; that enough alcohol will weaken all inhibitory associations; that the law of frequency will be apparently suspended in the delirium of fever or even in ordinary sleep; that the capacity for intellectual achievement may be weakened by disease of the thyroid gland; that a child's temperament or disposition will suffer complete change during an attack of indigestion. This caution not to forget the real and frequent influence of direct physiological changes in the nervous system upon human intellect and character ought perhaps to be repeated at the beginning of every chapter from now on. But I shall entrust to the reader the duty of remembering it for himself.

CHAPTER XV

The Connections Between Sense Stimuli and Mental States: Connections of Impression

§ 42. *Inborn and Acquired Connections of Impression*

Inborn Connections. — Every educated person knows that some sort of connection exists between events taking place in the physical world and his mental states; that he hears sounds because there are sound-waves, and smells odors when certain gases are present in the atmosphere. The immediate connection is between the action of neurones in the brain and the mental states; but since these neurones are aroused to action by afferent neurones from the sense organs, and since these afferent neurones are aroused by the physical event either directly or through some physiological process, we commonly speak of the total series of connections between the physical event and the mental state as one connection.

Such connections are due to inborn capacities. Sound waves of 50-100 vibrations per second arouse a feeling of a low tone and those of 10,000-20,000 vibrations per second arouse a feeling of a high tone, simply because man's mind is so constituted by nature that they do. Ether vibrations make us feel reds and greens and blues while rapid molecular motion makes us feel warm, just because these forms of connection have been established by natural evolution.[1] Given a certain physical stimulus and a certain feeling follows.

Acquired Connections.—At first thought this seems to be the end of the matter; but, as was briefly stated in Chapter II, § 8, *the stimulus itself is not the sole cause of the mental state.* To the question, "What determines what things anyone feels at any moment?" common sense gives the ready answer, "That which is there to be sensed, —to be seen, heard or touched." But common sense is only partly right. The physical stimulus affecting the sense organs is one, but only one, of the causes which determine what the percept shall be. For (1) we may feel different things, have different percepts, from the same stimulus; moreover (2) we may have the same percept from different stimuli; and in the third place (3) we may feel a thing when there is no physical stimulus corresponding to it.

Thus (1) the same cup of coffee tastes sweet after quinine and bitter after honey; the same light is bright by night and dim by day; the same gray looks reddish on a green background and greenish on a red background. The same air waves which make me feel a vague tumult of sound, make the musician feel the tones of five distinct instruments combined in a harmony; the same mass of colors is a blur to me and a definite group of micro-organisms to the trained microscopist.

Thus (2) patches of quite different shades may all be

[1]There is no absolute necessity that the connections should be as they are. Man might conceivably have been such a creature that sound waves of 50-100 vibrations would make him feel cold and those of 20,000-40,000 vibrations make him feel warm. There might conceivably exist connections between the pressure of the X-rays and feelings of some sort unlike any we now possess. Or we might lack, as the fishes apparently and as some lower animals certainly do, any connections between sound waves and mental states. The existing connections represent only one of many possible arrangements.

felt as the same green (*e.g.*, grass in the sunshine and in the shade); the table top is felt to be a rectangle, though seen as a sharp rhombus; in a brief glance at the letters 'bad oratory,' half an audience saw the same word as when the letters presented were 'laboratory;' so also with 'peneil' and 'pencil.'

Thus (3) occasionally in waking hours, and customarily in dreams, we see and hear and smell and taste things though neither they nor anything like them is present.

Not only the outside stimulus, but also the inner constitution of the individual's mental life, decides what thing shall be felt. There is more to perception than passive impressibility by external forces. Every act of perception is really an act of association. What is felt depends not only upon how the afferent neurones are stimulated, but also upon what neurones they in turn arouse; not only upon what the external object is, but also upon (A) the past experiences and (B) the present tendencies of the individual who perceives it.

(A) The musician feels the sounds made by the string quintette differently from the untrained person, because he has in the past attended to musical sounds and learned to discriminate the parts of a harmony; the audience saw peneil as pencil because the pen il had so often connected with the thought pencil in their previous reading. (B) The coffee tastes now sweet, now bitter, the light is now bright, now dim, according to the backgrounds of taste and illumination accompanying them; the 'bad oratory' was felt as 'laboratory' because in the minds of the audience (a class seated in a laboratory where they had been doing laboratory work for the month past) the thought of laboratory was especially ready to be aroused, was in a line of little resistance. If 'laboratory' had been shown for a fraction of a second to an audience accustomed to listening to and thinking about speeches, many of them would have seen it as 'bad oratory.'

§ 43. *The Law of Association in the Case of Connections of Impression*

In General.—What one feels at any given sense stimulus depends then upon what one has felt and upon what one is feeling at the time. Not only the mere capacities for responding to certain events in the physical world by feelings of certain qualities, but also the development of these capacities by training and their dependence upon the particular circumstances attending each case of response, must be taken into account in a study of the connections between sense stimuli and mental states. Nurture modifies nature even in the case of feelings from the senses. The connections between sense stimuli and mental states are partly instinctive and partly learned. Perception involves the influence of training and is explained by the law of association as surely as is the formation of habits; there are habits of perceiving as truly as there are habits of thought and conduct. The incoming stimulus from any set of afferent neurones may discharge into any one of several cell groups; which one it will arouse depends upon the general laws of association and assimilation deciding which connection is strongest.

In Detail.—Other things being equal the strongest connection will be (1) that favored by inborn structure, (2) that most frequently made, (3) the most recently made, (4) that with the most easily excitable mental state and (5) that most in harmony with the general set of the mind at the time. Illustrations of the influence of each of these factors may be found in anyone's daily experience. (1) is of course illustrated in every minute of perceptual experience. The trained nurse reading 'abominable' as 'abdominal' illustrates (2); the householder who, after a burglary at his house, heard every noise as a fumbling at the door illustrates a combination of (3) and (4). The psychology class who saw 'psychogaly' as 'psychology' illustrates (5) combined with (2) and (3). The author's name was heard by various people to whom he was introduced at the time of the discovery of gold in Alaska, as Klondike; and an old lady in a country town once greeted him as Mr. Corn-doctor.

One consequence of the laws of association and assimilation in the case of connections of impression is that any sense stimulus tends to be felt as some definite 'thing.' The incoming nerve currents have by the law of diffusion to go *somewhere* and the connections which have been made in the past are largely with cell actions corresponding to feelings of 'things.' So ink blots made at random often strike the observer as pictures of real objects; the clouds take on animal forms; there is a man in the moon; the wind in the trees is heard as a 'sighing.'

The Influence of the Law of the Mind's Set.— Three special forms of the influence of the general set of the mind, of the mental context in which the percept is felt, are so important as to deserve formulation as special laws. The first and most general is the *Law of Relativity,* that any stimulus will be felt, not as it would be if by itself alone, but in comparison with the sensations and percepts which accompany or precede it. Thus a gray on a black background will look whiter than when on a white background; a one-pound weight added to a pound will be felt as an increase, but will not when added to a hundred pounds. The second and third laws refer to special cases of the law of relativity. The *Law of Diminishing Returns* from increases in the amount of a stimulus (Weber's law) is that the same stimulus will produce a more intense sensation when added to a weak stimulus than when added to a strong one. Under this law belongs the case of the pound weight. Similarly an inch more makes 2 inches perceptibly longer, but adds little feeling of length to ten feet; it is easy to distinguish a three candle power lamp from a two candle power lamp, but between a two hundred and three and a two hundred and two candle power lamp practically no difference can be felt. The *Law of Contrast* is that one sensation or percept felt with or after another tends to take on the quality opposite to or complementary to that other. When the other is felt with it, we have *Simultaneous Contrast;* when the other is felt before it, we have *Successive Contrast.* Thus the gray on a black looks whiter and on a white blacker than it would by itself; a candle light looks brighter in the dark than in daylight; a tone seems lower after a high than after a low one; lemonade tastes sweeter after vinegar than after honey; a gray on red looks greenish; on blue, yellowish; and on green, reddish.

Percepts, Illusions and Hallucinations.—It follows from the facts so far stated that the same general process causes percepts, illusions and hallucinations. When the word beautiful is spoken and heard, hearing it is called a percept; when *dutiful* is spoken but *beautiful* heard, hearing it is called an illusion; when nothing is spoken (as in a dream) but beautiful is heard, hearing it is called an hallucination. In all three cases the same final brain process was aroused, the difference being that in the first case one afferent process excited it, in the second a slightly different process, and in the third no afferent process at all but some inner connection. In other words, when the sense stimulus present is the one that ordinarily arouses the mental fact, it is a case of perception; when the sense stimulus present is one that ordinarily arouses some other mental fact, it is illusion; and when the sense stimulus is *nil*, it is hallucination.

What is commonly called perception is a mixture of perception, illusion and hallucination. Thus in reading, some of the words which we feel ourselves to see are not seen at all and others are seen as quite different from their actual printed forms. There are misspellings in almost every book, but they pass unnoticed, unseen by the mental eye. Parts of words, even whole words, are often not present as sensory stimuli at all, the mind making them up out of whole cloth. So also in listening to spoken language we hear words which the ear does not hear at all. If one says rapidly in the proper context 'What time tis it?' or 'Please pass me ge butter,' the error will often be undetected. The letter t is often pronounced as d in such words as ability, certainty, falsity,[1] but only experts in phonetics notice the fact. Again and again in rapid speech words are totally omitted without anyone being the wiser.

§ 44. *The Control of Connections of Impression*

What is called the education of the senses and training in observation might better be called training in *acquiring associations* with sense stimuli. The difference between the untrained and the trained observer lies not in the action of the sense organs but in the previous experience which interprets their messages. The professional tester of tea has not a different tongue but a different set of experiences, a different stock of associations with various

[1] Where the t is far removed from the accented syllable.

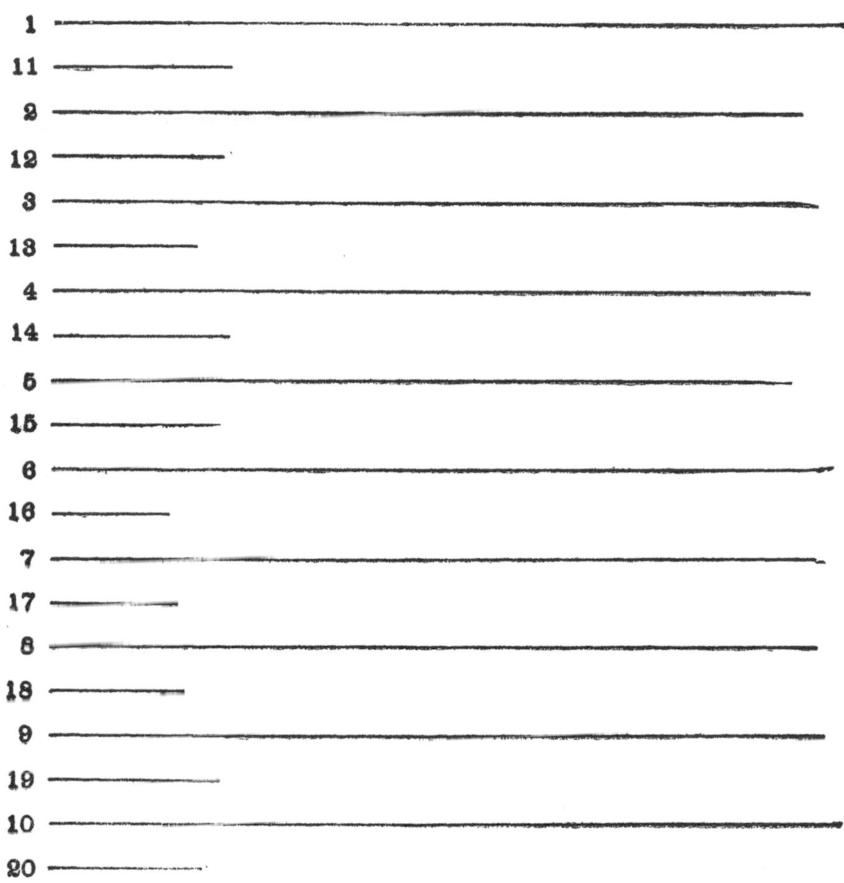

Fig. 76.

stimuli. The man of science sees more in the specimen because he knows more about it. One does not learn to see by perpetual staring, but by connecting each sight with knowledge about the thing seen. To educate the senses means (1) to form habits of systematic rather than hap-hazard examination, (2) to learn to recognize elements in complexes by first getting used to them singly, and (3) to connect each sensory stimulus with a separate identifiable feeling and with knowledge of its properties.

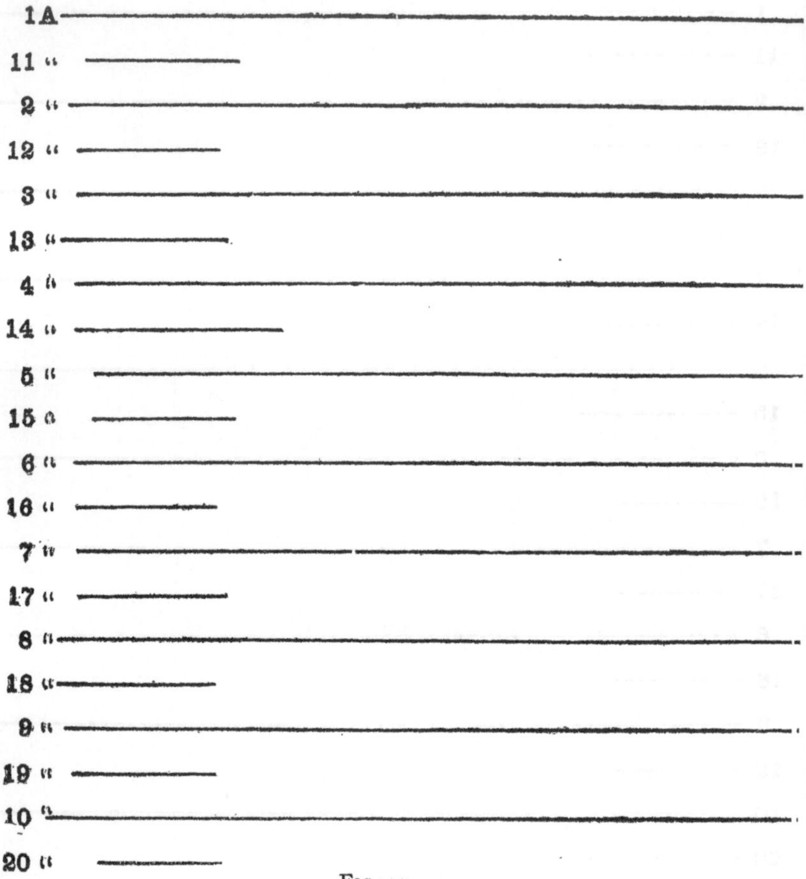

1 A
11 "
2 "
12 "
3 "
13 "
4 "
14 "
5 "
15 "
6 "
16 "
7 "
17 "
8 "
18 "
9 "
19 "
10 "
20 "

FIG. 77.

Exercises

1. Read again § 8 and recall the results of the experiment there described.

2. Illustrate individual differences in the capacities to feel things and qualities in response to sensory stimuli.

3. Illustrate individual differences in perception due to differences in previous experience.

4. Illustrate the law of diminishing returns in the case of the perception of movements. Of tastes.

5. Classify the following illusions as (A) those caused by

the strength of previous habit and (B) those caused by the temporary set of the mind:—

a. "An officer who superintended the exhuming of a coffin rendered necessary through a suspicion of crime, declared that he already experienced the odor of decomposition, though it was afterwards found that the coffin was empty." (Quoted from Carpenter's *Mental Physiology* by J. Sully in *Illusions* p. 108.)

b. "I never feel sure after wiping the blades of my skates, that they are perfectly dry, since they always seem more or less damp to my hand." (Sully.)

c. "If we are seated in a railway train which is quite stationary and watch through the window a train passing ours on a neighboring track, we feel our own train to be in motion in the opposite direction.

d. "I remember one night in Boston, whilst waiting for a 'Mount Auburn' car to bring me to Cambridge reading most distinctly that name upon the signboard of a car on which (as I afterward learned) North Avenue was painted." (James.)

6. Hold one hand in hot and the other in cold water for a few seconds; then put them both in the same dish of tepid water. Compare the feelings of the two hands.

Experiment 19. Color Contrast.—Take 5 pieces of the same gray paper. Lay them on sheets of white, black, red, green and blue paper. Cover with very thin tissue paper. Compare the five grays.

Take two pieces of the same green paper. Lay one on a red background, the other on a background of its own color. Cover as before and compare the two greens. Do similarily with red on a green and on a red background.

Experiment 20. The Law of Diminishing Returns.—(a) Look at line No. 1 of Fig. 76 then at line No. 1A of Fig. 77. Is the latter shorter or longer than No. 1. (Do not measure, judge by the eye alone.) Compare similarly lines 11 and 11A, 2 and 2A, etc., recording each judgment. After the 20 judgments have been recorded measure the lines and compare the frequency of right judgments in the case of lines 1-10 with that in the case of lines 11-20.

(b) On a sheet of paper 10 inches or more wide rule five lines 20, 40, 60, 80 and 100 millimeters long respectively. Place beside it a similar sheet and draw lines as nearly equal to the models

16

as you can without measuring or superposition. Do the same thing with another sheet, and continue until you have 10 sheets, each with five lines as nearly equal to the original models as you can draw them. Find, by measuring, the error made in each of the fifty lines. Compare the amount of the error for the 20 mm. line with that for the 40 mm. line and so on through the series.

Experiment 21. The Law of Association in Perception.— Print in the same style and size each of the following words upon a slip of paper and paste on a card about 3½ by 1½ inches: (1) good, (2) boy, (3) house, (4) pasent, (5) scarf, (6) sdirt, (7) chipon, (8) feather, (9) tackle, (10) tooch drwn, (11) genuine,

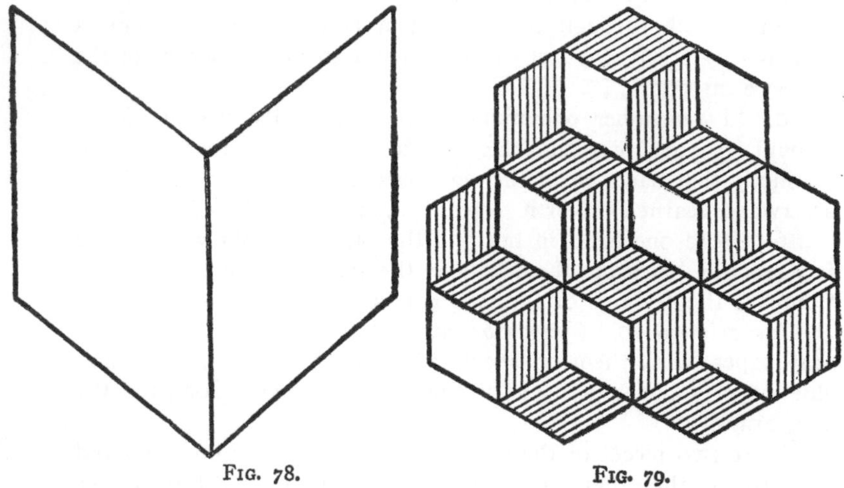

FIG. 78. FIG. 79.

(12) meawing, (13) reaeoning, (14) initate, (15) stoie, (16) morning, (17) frequmtly, (18) constant, (19) embrarderg.

Expose each (in the order given above) for one or two tenths of a second to some one unacquainted entirely with the cards or the object of the experiment, and have him write down what he sees in each case. Explain so far as you can the percepts felt. Compare the records of men and women in the case of words 6, 7, 9, 10, 15, and 19.

Experiment 22. Look at Fig. 78. Does it seem to be (1) a folded sheet with the folded edge toward you, or (2) a folded sheet with the folded edge away from you, or (3) a group of lines on a flat surface? Continue looking at it steadily. What happens? Make it seem like (1) (without altering the figure itself at all). Make it seem like (2). What do you do to make it seem like (1)? Shut your eyes; imagine a sheet of cardboard with the folded edge away from you, open your eyes and look at the figure. Which was it like, (1), (2) or (3)? Make it seem like (3). Which appearance is hardest to obtain: (1), (2) or (3)?

Experiment 23. How many blocks are there in Fig. 79? Continue looking at it steadily. What happens?

Experiment 24. How many different appearances can you

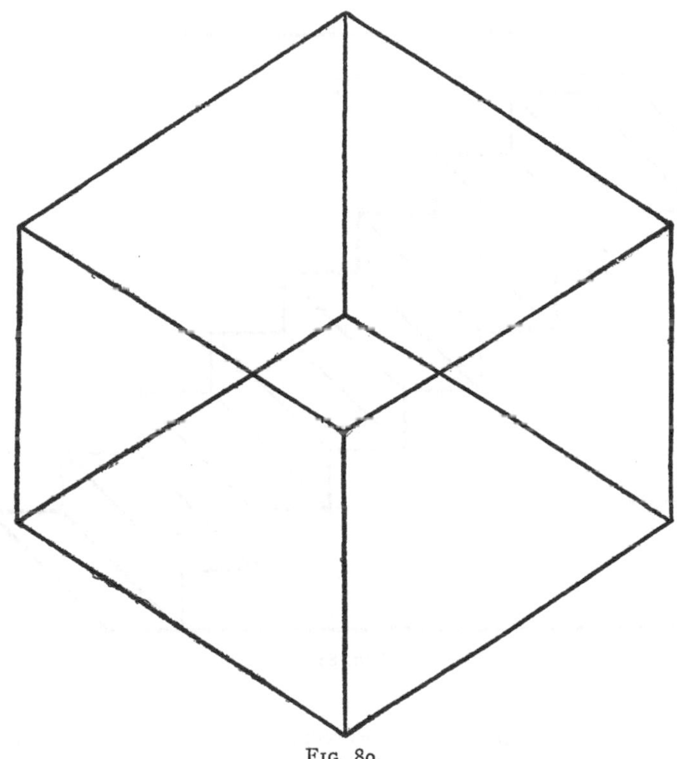

FIG. 80.

get from Fig. 80? Describe each of them. Why does it seem like an object of three dimensions rather than of two only, when it really is all in one plane?

Experiment 25. How many different appearances can you get from Fig. 81? Describe each of them. Which is the easiest to get and retain? Why?

7. In what other experiments have you found the alternation

of one impression with another in somewhat the same way as happens in Experiment 22.

8. Illustrate from your record of Experiment 22 the statement: "What thing is perceived will depend upon past experience."

9. Illustrate similarly; "What thing is perceived will depend upon the state of mind at the time of perceiving."

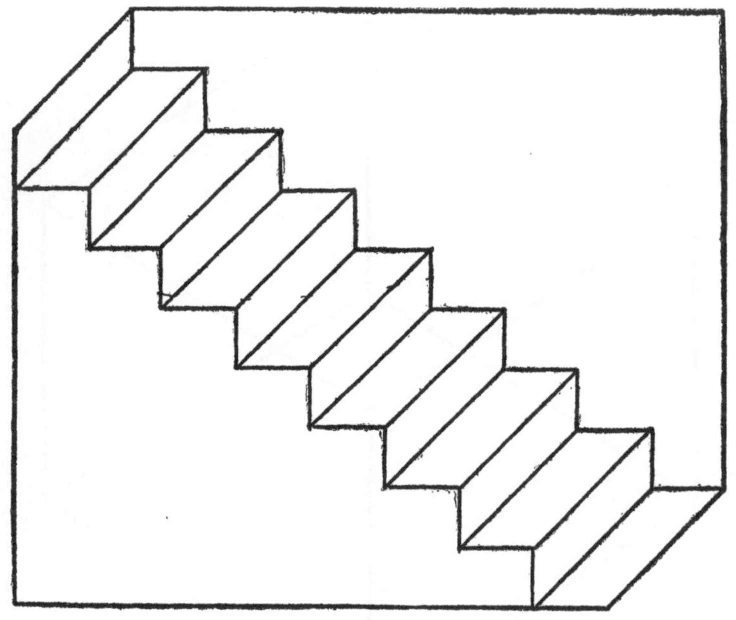

Fig. 81.

10. Illustrate similarly; "Perception is of definite and probable things."

11. Illustrate similarly the influence of frequency of connection in determining what percept a given sense stimulus will arouse.

12. From your records of Experiments 19 to 25 gather all the facts you can in support of any statements made in this chapter.

Arrange these facts in lists, each under the statement which it supports.

References

A. James, *Briefer Course*, II. (17-27), XX. (316-334).
Stout, *Manual*, 125-140, 199-209.
Titchener, *Outline*, §§ 27-30.

B. Ebbinghaus, *Grundzüge*, §§ 44-47.
James, *Principles*, XVII. (9-31), XIX. (82-133).
Wundt, *Physiologische Psychologie*, IX., XII.-XV.

CHAPTER XVI

The Connections Between one Mental State and Another

§ 45. *Associations of Ideas*

The Problem Stated.—The problem of this section may be stated in several ways. Given any mental state not due to a sense stimulus, how came it to be present? Given any mental state, what other mental state will it call up? What in addition to sense stimuli determines the order of our thoughts? What laws account for the ways in which mental states are connected among themselves? These four questions are substantially the same.

The first member of the connection, *i.e.,* the mental state that calls up, may be termed the antecedent, the stimulant or simply Thought 1; the second member of the connected pair, *i.e.,* the mental state that is called up, may be termed the consequent, sequent, resultant or simply Thought 2. Thought 1 may be a mental state of any sort; but Thought 2 cannot be a sensation or percept or any feeling that results directly from a sense stimulus, for then the connection would necessarily be not mental-mental, but physical-mental. Thought 2 is generally, perhaps always, an image, a feeling of meaning or intellectual relationship, or a judgment.

The complex states of mind which we ordinarily experience are the results of both the antecedent thought and of sense stimuli; a man does not often have a series of mental states due to purely mental connections. What he sees and hears, the feelings of his own body, and other sensory stimuli, color his thoughts and may redirect them. Still in day dreams, in serious thought on intellectual problems and in the flow of undisturbed memories, when little attention is paid to the physical world and to the warmth or cold or pain or movements of the body, the course of thought is almost exclusively explainable as the result of purely mental connections. And in any case we can study the influence of the present *thought* in determining the future apart from that of the sense stimuli which are also acting.

The General Law of Association in the Case of Purely Mental Connections.—Probably none of the purely mental connections are inborn, unlearned. Nature does not apparently provide any ready-made apparatus for such connections as thinking of six when one thinks of three and three. Our rich inheritance of connections between sense stimuli and mental states, sense stimuli and acts, and mental states and acts, is in sharp contrast to our utter poverty with respect to connections between one mental state and another. Nature gives only the general capacity to form such connections as soon as images, feelings of meaning and judgments have been acquired. One important result of the fact that all purely mental connections are due to nurture is that there is far less uniformity among human beings in the mental-mental than in the physical-mental connections. Light rays of a certain vibration-rate produce in seeing persons the feeling of red with comparatively small variations, but the sight of the color will arouse in one the thought of *red,* in another of *roth,* in another of *rouge,* in another of *corado,* according to the connections which have been acquired.

The mode of acquisition of the purely mental connections is by the action of the general law of association. The most frequent reason why one mental state calls up the thought of a certain object is that it *has been* its antecedent in our previous experience. Thinking of 6 times 7 makes us think of 42, because in school the 6 times 7 was deliberately connected with 42. The child thinks of the word dog as a sequent to the percept of the animal because he has heard and said the word in response to that percept before. All associations between percept of thing and name, percept of relation and name, percept of image of thing and class-name, between sensation and adjective, and the like, are clearly due to this law. Consider also the vast number of mental connections which owe their origin to arithmetical tables, paradigms and definitions learned, to books read, to sights seen and sounds heard in sequence. Throughout life we put one thing after another in order that the thought of the first may call up the thought of the second. The mental connections which attract our notice do so often by their very abnormality and rareness and so give a false notion of connections in general. For once that a thought calls up some unlikely sequent, there are a hundred times that it calls up the object which the law of association would lead us to expect. The law of association applied to the formation of purely mental connections may be roughly stated as follows: *Any mental state will be followed by that mental state by which it has been followed in the past.* A fuller statement of the law will be made later after certain apparent exceptions to it have been examined.

The Law of Partial Activity.—It is impossible to explain the following connections, which represent a very common sort, by the fact of Thought 1 having been followed by Thought 2 in the past:—

Case A. Thought 1. Of a large piece of ice in a cup of iced tea.
Thought 2. Of the ice trust.

Case B. Thought 1. I have lots of curiosity.
Thought 2. Of Eve.

In these and similar cases the first thought as a whole has surely never before gone with the second thought. But they are nevertheless to be explained by the law of association, for although Thought 1 has never been followed by Thought 2 in either case, a *part* of it has. In Case A the image or word *ice* is the only element of the total thought that is active in making the connection; in Case B the thought of curiosity is the active element. 'Ice—Ice trust' and 'Curiosity—Eve' are readily explainable by the law of association. In the total thought some one element frequently, indeed usually, will be thus active. The law should therefore be amended so as to read: *Any mental state will be followed by that mental state by which it or some part of it has been followed in the past.*

A Mental State Calls Up Its Previous Accompaniments.—There remain still some apparently unexplained cases such as the following:

Case A. Thought 1. Percept of Mr. S. reciting.
Thought 2. Image of Mr. S. at luncheon the day before.

Case B. Thought 1. Percept of the moon.
Thought 2. Image of a lamp with a round globe at home.

Here, as before, only a part of Thought 1 is operative, but the part acts not by calling up something which has *followed* it, but something which has been *simultaneous* with it and of which it was a part. The feeling of Mr. S. in the total of 'Mr. S. reciting' calls up the feeling of Mr. S. in the total of 'Mr. S. at luncheon.' The feeling of bright roundness in the total, 'bright roundness up in the sky there,' calls up the total, 'bright roundness of globe with rest of lamp.' It is a fact that mental states connect not only with their previous sequents but also with their previous accompaniments. Association is not only in a forward but also in a sideways direction. The law should read, 'by which it or some part of it has been followed *or accompanied.*'

Purely Mental Connections in General.—The facts of mental connections so far presented may be represented by easy symbols as follows:—

Let x be a total thought composed of the elements A B C
" y " " " " " " " " D E F
" z " " " " " " " " G H I
" v " " " " " " " " J K L
" w " " " " " " " " A M N

Let x have been followed by y
" A " " " " z
" x " " accompanied by v

Then x may call up y because y has followed x in the past.
Or x " " z " z " " a part of x in the past.
Or x may call up v because v has accompanied x in the past.
Or x may call up w because the elements M N have accompanied a part of x in the past.

Cases where Thought 1 as a whole leads to Thought 2 are called cases of *Total Recall;* cases where a part of Thought 1 leads to Thought 2 are called cases of *Partial Recall;* cases where some one element or feature of Thought 1 leads to Thought 2 are called cases of *Focal Recall.* These names are not well chosen; for they would, according to the common use of language, mean that all or part or a little *was recalled;* they should mean of course that all or a part or a little of a thought is active *in recalling.* Perhaps *Total, Partial* and *Very Partial Activity* would be more useful names. *Focal Activity* is only the extreme of partial activity.

Cases of partial or focal activity in which the recalling elements are present not only in Thought 1 but also in Thought 2, cases, that is, of the x w type, used to be called cases of *Association by Similarity.* In such cases Thought 1 and Thought 2 will of course be more or less similar, because one or more elements are the same in both, but they are not connected by their similarity. Mere similarity in and of itself has no tendency to result in connection. The thought of a red brick does not make us keep on thinking of red bricks.

The name *Association by Contiguity* has been used, first to denote connections between things which exist together in time or space, and later to denote all connections of the x y or x z or x v types. The name has outlived its usefulness.

The names (1) *Persistent* and (2) *Desistent* associations have been used[1] for (1) cases where the first thought or part of it remains and is an element in the sequent thought and (2) cases where it does not.

I have spoken of connections between one mental state and another and of connections between the thought of one thing and the thought of another thing, as if the two phrases meant the same. They really do not; quite different mental states may each be the thought of the same thing. Thus in the following connections the second members are in both cases the thought of George Eliot's novels, but they are different mental states :—

A. Thought 1. Adam Bede.
" 2. I like George Eliot's novels.

[1] By Professor M. W. Calkins.

B. Thought 1. Adam Bede.
" 2. I dislike George Eliot's novels.

If the student will notice his own trains of thought he will soon conclude that one mental state rarely calls up exactly the mental state which has in the past followed it. Suppose mental state A to be followed by mental state B; suppose that later A recurs. The emotional tone, the feelings of the accompanying circumstances, the general setting which composed in large measure mental state B, will in all probability not recur, but only the object or fact felt as the core of B. For instance, 'amo, amas, amat' is followed originally by the feeling, 'amamus; I am sick of this; how hot it is!' etc.; but 'amo, amas, amat' in my mind to-day calls up only the word 'amamus;' the setting it has, if any, is furnished by present circumstances. In short what is called up in Thought 2 is some object or fact. Just how the object is felt or the fact regarded is decided by present circumstances rather than by the way the object and fact were felt and regarded in the past when connected with Thought 1. The reason for this is that the settings of the object or fact in its original appearances were due largely to the sensory stimuli then active, and were different at different times. In recall (1) the sensory stimuli of the present far outweigh any images of the setting of earlier appearances, and (2) such images mutually interfere because of their unlikeness.

The Causes in Partial Activity.—The next step in an account of mental connections is to explain which part of Thought 1 will in cases of partial activity be operative in calling up the coming thought. It will, other things being equal, be that part which is attended to, which is interesting, which is held in the mind's focus. Just as of what the eyes see at any time, only the part that is in the center of the visual field arouses a clear percept; so of what is thought at any time, only the focal part will arouse the next idea. The other things that must be equal are all those which make one brain process more likely to discharge than another, such as conditions of nutrition, blood supply, fatigue and the like. About these little is known, but they are so effective as to prevent a psychologist from prophesying with any approach to certainty what part of any total thought will count in determining the next thought. If a school boy thinks, 'Christmas comes on December 25th,' he will in the long run be reminded of gifts, good things to eat and festivities, rather than of 'square root,' 'what is the etymology of December,' or 'December has 31 days;' the element *Christmas* being active rather than the element *25th* or *December.* But on any one occasion these or other features of the total thought may chance to be the determining factor of the next thought.

The Causes that Determine Which One of Several Possible Facts Shall be Called Up.—The account of mental connections so far given is adequate to explain why any mental state or part of a mental state calls up the idea which has gone with it. But any antecedent may have been followed by several different ideas. In such cases *which one* will be called up? Horse has gone with wagon, whip, harness, mane, car, barn, stall, etc. Which of these former associates will be the sequent in any given case when horse is thought of? The details of the general law of association contain the answer. The connection will be along the line of least resistance. The line of least resistance will be determined by the frequency, recency, vividness and resulting satisfaction of the connection, and the excitability of the sequent ideas.

Resulting satisfaction plays here a comparatively unimportant part directly for the reason stated in § 35 that in itself one image, feeling of meaning or judgment is little less or more pleasant than another. Horse-wagon, horse-whip, horse-harness, are as feelings alike indifferent. Resultant satisfaction is probably a partial explanation of the frequency of rhyming associations and the connection of certain epithets with things. The pleasure in the rhyme or in the fitness of the epithet may fix the two members of the connection firmly together so that the one will later call the other up. Indirectly, in the guidance of the process of association, as in schools, resulting satisfaction and discomfort are prime causes.

Frequency of connection in the past is the commonest cause of connection in the future. Thus the sight of a horse is almost sure to call up the word horse, no matter what else it may call up; 4×9 is, in an educated mind, almost sure o produce the thought of 36 if it has any sequent. In all cases where the feeling of a thing or quality calls up its name, where the sight of printed letters calls up the auditory or motor image of a word; where a word in one language calls up its translation in another; where familiar signals, such as the striking of a clock, calls up their corresponding events, and in many more,—frequency is the cause. No further illustrations are needed; they may be found in the trains of thought appearing in connection with almost every example in arithmetic done, every page read, every hour of daily life.

That the recency of a connection between one thought and another increases the probability that the first will call up the second also needs no proof and little comment. Anyone's mental life during any day will substantiate and illustrate the fact. The following are actual cases:—

A. Thought 1. The sight of some fruit.
    " 2. Mr. S. asked me this morning if I liked fruit.

B. Thought 1. Of Spanish wars.
" 2. Of the trouble [then arising] in China.
C. Thought 1. Of cable cars, horse cars and of my feet on the pavement.
" 2. Of cable cars just keeping up with a horse car yesterday — dreadfully slow.

That one thought which has gone with another in some vivid, intense experience will be more likely to call it up than to call up some other to which it led in the course of commonplace, unattended-to life is also proved and illustrated by everyone's experience. In the mind of the man who has dined with the king, every future meal will be honored by his majesty's presence in imagination. In 1901 the mention of the word anarchist called up in every mind the lamented death of President McKinley.

Every day life also sufficiently illustrates the fact that a half-awake, ready-to-be-excited idea, one due to some vivid and deep impression, is especially likely to be called up. We all know to our discomfort how easily the events of a trip to Europe are called up in our friends' minds; how everything will remind the doting mother of some saying or act of her child; how quickly conversation in the country store turns to the great event of the burning of Thomson's cow-barn.

Finally, to understand which of its former associates any mental state will call up we need to bear constantly in mind the caution of page 167. It was there stated that the action of the brain at any time must not be considered as a definite action of a limited number of neurones and nothing more, but as such definite, special, emphatic action plus more or less action in a whole system of neurones, even throughout the entire nervous system.

The nature of this more general action or 'set' of entire systems might be, we then saw, an important factor in determining into what neurones the specially active neurone group would discharge.

This fact implies concerning the connections between one mental state and another that which thought any given thought will call up of the many that it might call up, will be determined in part by the general trend of thought at the time, the general frame or set of mind one is in, the general system of ideas which is as a whole more or less aroused and ready to appear. For example, if it is vacation time and I am digging in my garden and a neighbor leans over the fence and says, "What do you think of James?" I shall probably think, "What James?" If I were in a class room in the university and a student asked the same question, I should think of the gifts and work of the eminent psychologist.

The same thought may arouse different associates according to whether it is felt in one's work system or play system, one's week day or Sunday system; at home or at school; by oneself or among others; in one's scientific or one's sentimental system; in the mood of elation or of depression. Besides these great systems there are multitudes of lesser systems, each exerting its influence on the direction of thoughts that occur within it. Notice how every new thought in the following reverie is due, not to the previous thought alone, but also to the general system of 'African war affairs:'—

"Sensation of getting warm under sun while walking fast.
Soldiers in Africa compared with me.
My bag not like soldier's gun but officer's sword.
Officers do not wear swords, but I saw a picture of one with a scabbard recently.
British have learned a lot this war.

Boers taught officers to quit wearing swords by shooting at officers.
Old chivalric notions dying out of warfare; thought of Fontenoy and the silly exchange of courtesies.
Newspaper tale that Roberts has society men on his staff as well as real men.
Does he have to?
That's why he keeps ahead of Kitchener, by not appearing harsh.
What's Kitchener doing as chief of staff?
Roberts sending him to relieve Rushenburg, something like sending him to the Victoria West District.
I guess they work separately better than together.
I would better think of something useful.
I'll work up this train of thought."

The action of the general law of association in the case of connections between one mental state and another may be summarized as follows: *Any fact thought of will call up that fact, the thought of which has accompanied or followed it or a part of it most frequently, most recently, in the most vivid experience and with the most resultant satisfaction, and which is most closely connected with the general set of mind at the time.*

The physiological basis of this law is simply that of the general law of association, the neural connections being in this case between associative neurones. The connections between the thought of one object and that of another illustrate the general law of the transmission of the nervous impulse along the line of least resistance or closest connection.

Individual Differences in Purely Mental Connections.—Individuals differ tremendously in the number of purely mental connections which they possess and in the time required to make the connection. What is commonly called knowledge is, in psychological terms, *mental connections,* error equalling *incorrect connections* and ignorance the *absence of connections.* As people differ in the amount of information possessed, so roughly they differ in the number of purely mental connections. The differences are then obviously tremendous. Individual differences in the case of the time it takes for one idea to call up another have been proved to exist by actual measurement. Even among so-called 'normal' children the range is such that some children require more than twice as long for the same process. If so-called deficient children are included the differences are much more pronounced.

Before leaving this general discussion of the laws of the connections between the thought of one object and the thought of another, I may refer the reader to the warning given in § 41. Ideas occasionally, even often, come up which are highly improbable so far as frequency, recency, vividness, and so on are concerned, and which can be attributed only to some at present unaccountable disturbance of the nervous system,—some process of inner change that is beyond our ken. In sleep, fevers and mania this is perhaps the rule.

Exercises

1. How does the following anecdote illustrate the general fact that any idea will call up that idea which has gone with it or a part of it?

Six gentlemen, all unacquainted each with the others, had been conversing in a railway carriage. One offered to tell the profession of each of the others, provided they answer one apparently irrelevant question. They agreed. "He drew five leaves from his note-book, wrote a question on each, and gave one to each of his companions with the request that he write the answer below. When the leaves were returned to him, he turned, after reading them, without hesitation to the others, and said to the first, 'You are a man of science'; to the second, 'You are a soldier'; to the third, 'You are a philologer'; to the fourth, 'You are a journalist'; to the fifth, 'You are a farmer'. All admitted that he was right, whereupon he got out and left the five behind. Each wished to know what question the others had received; and behold, he had given the same question to each. It ran thus: 'What being destroys what it has itself brought forth?'

To this the naturalist had answered, 'vital force'; the soldier, 'war'; the philologist, 'Kronos'; the publicist, 'revolution'; the farmer, 'a boar'." (H. Steinthal, *Einleitung in die Psychologie und Sprachwissenschaft,* pp. 166-167; quoted in James', *Principles of Psychology,* vol. II., p. 108.)

2. Arrange the connections given below in three groups according to the amount of Thought 1 that is active in calling up Thought 2.

A. Thought 1. Seeing a wrought-iron letter-rack on the breakfast table.
Thought 2. I thought, 'That has been made by a student in the manual training class.'

B. Thought 1. 2 of A.
" 2. What is the value of manual training?

C. " 1. 2 of B.
" 2. Men engaged in education are now looking to the *practical* in life.

D. Thought 1. Thought of my physician.
" 2. " " his asking me to study medicine.

E. " 1. 2 of D.
" 2. Thought of my replying that I was afraid of contagious diseases.

F. " 1. 3×9.
" 2. 27.

G. " 1. A noun is the name......
" 2. ....of a thing.

3. What per cent. of the connections in each of the following passages exemplify total or nearly total activity of the antecedent thought? Can you recall other quotations showing the same difference? In what sort of intellects are mental connections made by the total or nearly total activity of the antecedent?

I. "'But where could you hear it?' cried Miss Bates. 'Where could you possibly hear it, Mr. Knightley? For it is not five minutes since I received Mrs. Cole's note—no, it cannot be more than five—or at least ten—for I had got my bonnet and spencer on, just ready to come out—I was only gone down to speak to Patty again about the pork—Jane was standing in the passage—were you not, Jane?—for my mother was so afraid that we had not any salting-pan large enough. So I said I would go down and see, and Jane said: "Shall I go down instead? for I think you have a little cold, and Patty has been washing the kitchen." "Oh, my dear," said I—well, and just then came the note. A Miss Hawkins—that's all I know—a Miss Hawkins, of Bath. But, Mr. Knightley, how could you possibly have heard it? for the very moment Mr. Cole told Mrs. Cole of it, she sat down and wrote to me. A Miss Hawkins—' " (Jane Austen, "*Emma*," quoted by James, *Principles of Psychology,* vol. I, p. 571.)

II. "She always was clever," said poor Mrs. Nickleby, brightening up, "always from a baby. I recollect when she was only two years and a half old, that a gentleman who used to visit very much at our house—Mr. Watkins, you know, Kate, my dear, that your poor papa went bail for, who afterwards ran away to the United States, and sent us a pair of snow shoes, with such an affectionate letter that it made your poor dear father cry for a week. You remember the letter? In which he said that he was very sorry he couldn't repay the fifty pounds just then, because his capital was all out at interest, and he was very busy making his fortune, but that he didn't forget you were his god-daughter, and he should take it very unkind if we didn't buy you a silver coral and put it down to his old account? Dear me, yes, my dear, how stupid you are! and spoke so affectionately about the old port wine that he used to drink a bottle and a half of every time he came. You must remember, Kate."

"Yes, yes, mamma; what of him?"

"Why, that Mr. Watkins, my dear," said Mrs. Nickleby, slowly, as if she were making a tremendous effort to recollect something of paramount importance; "that Mr. Watkins—he wasn't any relation, Miss Knag will understand, to the Watkins who kept the Old Boar in the village; by the by, I don't remember whether it was the Old Boar or the George the Third, but it was one of the two, I know, and it's much the same—that Mr. Watkins said, when you were only two years and a half old, that you were one of the most astonishing children he ever saw. He did indeed, Miss Knag, and he wasn't at all fond of children, and couldn't have had the slightest motive for doing it. I know it was he who said so, because I recollect as well as if it was only yesterday, his borrowing twenty pounds of her poor dear papa the very moment afterwards." (*Nicholas Nickleby.*)

III. "To be, or not to be: that is the question:
Whether 'tis nobler in the mind to suffer
The slings and arrows of outrageous fortune,
Or to take arms against a sea of troubles,
And by opposing end them? To die: to sleep;
No more; and by a sleep to say we end
The heart-ache and the thousand natural shocks
That flesh is heir to, 'tis a consummation
Devoutly to be wish'd. To die, to sleep;
To sleep: perchance to dream; ay, there's the rub;
For in that sleep of death what dreams may come
When we have shuffled off this mortal coil,
Must give us pause: there's the respect
That makes calamity of so long life;
For who would bear the whips and scorns of time,
The oppressor's wrong, the proud man's contumely,
The pangs of despised love, the law's delay,
The insolence of office and the spurns
That patient merit of the unworthy takes,
When he himself might his quietus make
With a bare bodkin? who would fardels bear,
To grunt and sweat under a weary life,
But that the dread of something after death,
The undiscover'd country from whose bourn
No traveller returns, puzzles the will
And makes us rather bear those ills we have
Than fly to others that we know not of?"

IV. ......"Two beggars told me
I could not miss my way: will poor folks lie,
That have afflictions on them knowing 'tis
A punishment or trial? Yes; no wonder,
When rich ones scarce tell true. To lapse in fulness
Is sorer than to lie for need, and falsehood
Is worse in kings than beggars. My dear lord!
Thou art one o' the false ones. Now I think on thee,
My hunger's gone; but even before, I was
At point to sink for food. But what is this?
Here is a path to 't: 'tis some savage hold:

I were best not call; I dare not call: yet famine,
Ere clean it o'erthrow nature, makes it valiant.
Plenty and peace breeds cowards: hardness ever
Of hardiness is mother."

(*Cymbeline,* Act III., Scene VI.)

4. (a) Give two illustrations of connections of the X Y type (see page 242).
   (b) Give two illustrations of connections of the X Z type (see page 242).
   (c) Give two illustrations of connections of the X V type (see page 242).
   (d) Give two illustrations of connections of the X W type (see page 242).

5. (a) Which element of the total thought, 'Tuesday, election day, being a holiday, the stores will be closed,' would be most likely to be operative in calling up the next thought in the mind of a candidate for office? In the mind of a school boy? In the mind of a housekeeper?

   (b) Compose a similar illustration.

6. (a) Give three illustrations of one idea calling up a certain one of its previous associates because of the frequency of the connection. (b) Give three illustrations of the power of recency of connection. (c) Three of the power of vividness. Three of the power of membership in the same mental system.

7. Give the most probable causes for the connections which are shown by the following trains of thought. That is, state in the case of each connection whether the sequent was called up because it was the only connection or because it was the most frequent connection or because it was the most recent or because it was the most vivid, etc.

"I saw a paper which I had written for the course in philosophy.

I wondered whether the paper would be accepted.
Then I wondered what criticism I would get.
That reminded me that I must study my philosophy lesson.
Then I thought that the lesson was about Aristotle.
This reminded me that he was called the father of the sciences.
Then I thought about his logic.

This reminded me of Harris' treatment of logic in his 'Psychologic Foundations.'

By thinking of the word psychologic I thought of psychology.

Then I thought of the psychology class.

That reminded me that I had not yet written out any train of thought."

"Yesterday we received a letter from my sister who is off on a yachting trip. One of the men on board is a young fellow who is to be an assistant pastor in the fall. This brought up the church, and then came the school where I teach, which is just beside the church. This brought up one of my old pupils who is now in Germany. Then came an experience that my brother, who has just returned from India, told yesterday of being cheated in a bicycle tire by some German. The thought of my brother suggested India and I thought of some snake stories that he had told about that country. The snakes suggested something I had seen in the morning paper about some albino snakes at Bronx Park."

8. Looking in turn at each of the words printed below (keep all the later words covered by a card until the first, second and so on have been allowed to call up their associations) note and record the fact which it calls up. State the apparent cause for each of the connections made.

seven	dress
name	potato
dinner	game
friend	psychology
election	religion
instinct	river
house	fast
picture	Japan
association	easy
home	walking

§ 46. *Memory*

Memory and the Law of Association.—The terms memory and remember are used to refer to (1) the revival of a mental fact in imagination, (2) the revival of a fact plus the feeling of its having been in one's experience at some time in the past, (3) the revival of the appropriate mental fact in response to a situation, and (4) the revival of a movement or set of movements. The causes of the revival of movements will be stated in Chapter XVIII. The causes of the revival of mental facts are found in the general laws describing the formation and operation of connections between one mental state and another, the revival of mental facts being simply the result of the laws of the association of ideas.

The answer that has been given to the question, 'Given any mental state, what idea will be called up?', will answer also the question, 'What decides whether any mental fact shall reappear in memory?' The only need for a separate section on memory is that some new questions arise when the process of mental connection is studied from the point of view of the 'to be recalled fact' rather than from the point of view of the 'mental fact present.'

The probability of revival of any mental fact depends upon the strength of the original impression and the number of situations which lead to it. If fact A is impressed deeply, it will by the laws of intensity tend to be called up. If there are a hundred mental states which have led to fact A, it has by the law of association a hundred times the chance of being called up that it would have if there were only one mental state which had led to it.

To make sure that a mental fact will reappear, *e.g.*, that you do not forget to write a letter to Mr. A, you may either fix firmly the fact by attending to it, repeating it, etc.; or you may arrange so that many of the day's situations will call up the fact 'Write a letter to Mr. A,' *e.g.*, by saying to yourself: 'After dinner I must write to A. When I get home I must write to A. Before I go to bed I must write to A. Do nothing until A is written to.'

To recall a fact we try one after another those facts

which have gone with the desired fact in the hope that some one of them will call it up. Thus in trying to think of a certain man's name we think of the different occasions when we have seen and spoken to him, of the things he did, of the persons who also know and may have spoken of him, of his appearance and ways and the like, of names that we feel are like his name.

Appropriate Revival.—For practical purposes it is not the mere revival of a mental fact that counts but its revival at the proper situation. To recall this man's name is useless unless it is recalled at the sight of his face. To recall 1763 is useless unless it is recalled in connection with the Treaty of Paris or some other relevant fact. To recall 8:42 is useless unless it is recalled in connection with 'the train goes at.' Thus the problem of memory becomes still more similar to that of the association of ideas in general. In arranging for the revival of a mental fact, we commonly arrange for its connection with a particular situation. We try to make sure that 8 will be thought of *and thought of after 4+4;* that Shakspere will be thought of *and thought of with Hamlet, Lear and Othello.*

Goodness of memory depends upon the permanence of impressions, the permanence of connections, their number and their nature or arrangement. To have a first class memory one must retain for long the effects of an impression, must retain for long the effects of a connection, must have a goodly number of connections and must have things connected in logical, useful ways. It is better, for instance, to remember *amat* for a year than for a day and to keep the connection 'he loves is *amat*' for a year than for a day; to have a hundred such connections rather than one; to have fifty connections like he loves—amat, they love—amant, I love—amo, amabat—he was loving, amaverant—they had loved, rather than fifty like amo-amas, amas-amat, amat-amamus, amamus-amatis, amatis-amant, amant-amabam.

These facts are well illustrated in the stock methods of memorizing; *Repetition, Concentration* and *Recall.* Repetition strengthens both the impressions and the connection between them and is easy and natural, but is somewhat wasteful of time. Concentration, or prolonged attention to the fact to be remembered, strengthens the impressions and the connection between them and saves time, but at the expense of effort. Recall (*i.e.,* the expression *from within* of the fact to be remembered, after one or more impressions of it from without) gains the extra advantage of forming the connection in the way in which it will be required to act later[1] and is conceded to be the best method of the three.

The general permanence of impressions and connections, the mere retentiveness of the mind, is decided largely by original capacity and the general conditions of bodily health. The permanence of any particular impression or connection depends also upon the degree of attention given to it, its vividness, and the frequency of its repetition. The number of connections depends upon experience or training. The choice of logical and useful connections depends upon experience as directed by the capacity to see the essential elements in situations.

Individual Differences in Memory.—Individual differences in the power to remember are among the most striking found in mental life. For some it is a heavy burden to keep in mind the names of a hundred friends, the necessary detail of a single business or profession,

[1] The connection required is to think of B on seeing A; it is therefore more useful to practice 'see A think B' rather than 'see A see B.'

and perhaps a hundreth part of what is learned. For others there seems no need of more than a casual impression to fix a thing in memory. Of such a one James writes,

"He never keeps a written note of anything, yet is never at a loss for a fact which he has once heard. He remembers the old addresses of all his New York friends living in numbered streets, addresses which they themselves have long since moved away from and forgotten. He says that he should probably recognize an individual fly, if he had seen him thirty years previous—he is, by the way, an entomologist. As an instance of his desultory memory, he was introduced to a certain colonel at a club. The conversation fell upon the signs of age in man. The colonel challenged him to estimate his age. He looked at him, and gave the exact day of his birth, to the wonder of all. But the secret of this accuracy was that, having picked up some days previously an army-register, he had idly turned over its list of names, with dates of birth, graduation, promotions, etc., attached, and when the colonel's name was mentioned to him at the club, these figures, on which he had not bestowed a moment's thought, involuntarily surged up in his mind."[1]

These differences are due to (1) differences in the original capacity to retain impressions and connections, (2) differences in interest and (3) differences in the training of the capacity. The excellent memory for names as connected with faces so often found amongst clergymen and politicians is probably a case of interest. Names are attended to and thought over because of the professional interest in them. Many a woman of generally feeble memory can remember every dress she has owned since she was ten years old. The reason that men of poor general capacity to retain do as well as they do in the memory work of science, business and other walks

[1] *Principles of Psychology,* I, p. 661.

of life is apparently that they train themselves to learn facts in the most logical and useful ways and so get on with a little material well ordered.

Exercises

1. What means do you yourself take to make sure of remembering a fact? Explain why each is useful.

2. What fact probably explains both of the following cases?—

A young man knew by heart a large percentage of the products of every number up to a thousand by every number up to a thousand; he could give the population of hundreds of cities and counties. He did not remember names or poetry or miscellaneous facts much, if any, better than a person of moderately good memory.

An ignorant waiter, whose duty it was to care for hats and coats left at the door of a hotel dining room, is reported to have never made a mistake in years in recalling which hat belonged to which man of the hundreds who came to the hotel each day.

3. Which would be the better way to commit to memory a speech, to sit in one's chair and read it to oneself or to stand up, and say it out loud?

4. Find what evidence you can from your knowledge of yourself and of your acquaintances to support the following statements:—

(a) A good memory over a short interval does not imply a good memory over a long interval. (b) A good logical memory may go with a very poor verbal memory. (c) Very stupid people may have excellent memories.

§ 47. *The Control of Purely Mental Connections*

Habit Rules Thought.—If one desires to have one fact call up another, the two should be put together. The certainty of the recall will depend upon the frequency and vigor with which the two are put together. Thought like conduct is a matter of habit, and habits result only from painstaking connections. The intellect does not work logically or usefully of its own accord, but only by being practiced in or habituated to logical and useful associations of mental facts. For instance, the person cannot help becoming intellectually commonplace who habitually listens to and participates in such talk as: "I saw Mrs. Jones yesterday. She was going down town." "She told me she was going to buy a hat." "Yes, she showed it to me this morning. She said it cost twenty dollars." "I don't believe she paid cash. The Jones live away beyond their income." "Mr. Jones' health is not very good, I'm told; it would be very hard for them if he broke down." "It has been a terrible winter for sickness," etc., etc., etc.

Adult students who are by nature of a superior intellectual calibre and by training supplied with many useful systems of connections between facts, are prone to forget the bondage to purely habitual associations which masters less gifted and less mature minds. The following examples will help to make real the true state of affairs, and to emphasize the obvious but neglected practical rule: Put together facts which you wish to go together, and keep apart facts which you wish to be separate:—

Children are found to learn long division far more easily if in short division they are taught to put the line above or at the right of, instead of below, the dividend and the quotient above the line or to the right of it, thus: $4|\frac{422}{1688}$ or 4|1688|422. The reason is of course that they are saved the trouble of forming a new and contradictory set of associations when they begin long division.

Children taught the numbers from 1 to 20 and then from 20 to 40 or higher are found to have difficulty, after learning to write those from 20 to 40, in writing those from 13 to 19, although in their first learning they had had no trouble. The errors made are writing 61 for sixteen, 81 for eighteen and the like. The reason is that they form with the numbers above twenty the association of putting the digit denoted by the first part of the word first in order and the digit denoted by the second part of the word second in order. Thus thirty-eight is 38, twenty-six is 26. When now they hear sixteen or eighteen, they tend to follow the recent habit of making the order of digits the order of the syllables of the word.

Three quarters of a page of a magazine contained an advertisement of the Oneita Clothing. One quarter of it contained an advertisement of the Munsing Clothing. Many people sent to the Munsing Company orders for the Oneita Clothing.

Systems of Associations. — The arrangement of mental connections in useful systems adds greatly to their efficiency. Just as science orders the incoherent mass of experiences of the world at large, so any individual may, by having facts presented to him in coherent systems and by being encouraged to recall facts in a logical order, become a more efficient thinker.

The capacity to make connections with some element of the antecedent thought,—*i.e.*, the capacity for partial activity,—is on the whole more valuable than that for total activity. We should train ourselves to survey each fact and to select its essential element or feature to be the antecedent to the next thought. To learn the gist of a passage is thus often a more profitable task than to learn it verbatim.

Apart from inborn capacity the efficiency of a man's memory depends on his general health, the degree of attention he bestows on facts, the care with which he arranges them into systems, and the zeal with which he works over these facts, recalling them, comparing them and thinking about them. Any training which teaches us (1) to consider facts fully and thoughtfully, (2) to compare them, to put those together which belong together and to study their relationships, and (3) to recall them on all suitable occasions, so as to connect them with relevant facts of daily life, will improve memories so far as they are improvable.

References

A. James, *Briefer Course,* XVI. (253-271), XVIII.
Stout, *Manual,* 418-446.
Titchener, *Outline,* §§ 52-55.
B. Ebbinghaus, *Grundzüge,* §§ 60-64.
James, *Principles,* XIV., XVI. (653-689).
Wundt, *Physiologische Psychologie,* XIX. (§§ 1-4).

CHAPTER XVII

The Connections Between One Mental State and Another *(Continued)*

§ 48. *Purposive Thinking*

Purposive Thinking Equals Spontaneous Thinking Plus Selection.—We distinguish spontaneous or aimless thinking from controlled or purposive thinking. In the former ideas flow on at random, unchecked by any interference on the part of our general intentions and aiming at no desired goal. The prattle of babies, the reveries and haphazard trains of thought which come as we sit idly thinking of nothing in particular, and the majority of dreams are of this sort. In the latter some end is in view; our thoughts are kept so far as may be under control and make an intelligible sequence.

The connections in controlled thinking follow the same law as those in spontaneous thinking. The difference is that in controlled thinking each thought as it comes is attended to; its usefulness is judged in the light of our general system of ideas and purposes concerning the topic in hand; it is allowed to remain and influence the future course of thought only when it seems fit. So also of any total thought, that element which seems most useful to our purpose is definitely selected, attended to and encouraged to call up its connections. In spontaneous thinking we take whatever comes. In controlled thinking we select and reject in view of the goal we wish to attain.

This process of attentive consideration and selection or rejection is clearly shown in the search for a proper word to express a meaning, in attempts to solve problems of all sorts, from the simplest riddle or puzzle to the most abstruse question in mathematics or science, and in summoning evidence to support an argument. *E.g.*, you wish an adjective to describe a person who habitually enjoys what you do to entertain him, puts himself at your point of view and disagrees with nobody. You think: "Affable—no! that means more active effort at being pleasant—agreeable—no! agreeing would do better—appreciative—yes! but that doesn't include his readiness to accept almost any statement—compliant would mean that, but misses the appreciative, easily suited nature—complaisant—no! that isn't it at all—suitable—we ought to be free to use suitable to mean one who can be suited, can be pleased—pleasable is just it and isn't ambiguous. That's the word. He is a pleasable man."

The Process of Selection.—Selection and survival of the fit thoughts; inhibition and elimination of the unfit—these are the essentials of purposive thinking. The forces that select and inhibit are the feeling of approval or satisfaction and its opposite. The inhibition of the unfit thought is often accompanied by feelings of effort; often the unfit thought is banished only by voluntary attention to something else. Thoughts of play will intrude while the pupil is working out a problem in geometry, and their expulsion, or,—what is the same thing,—the persistence of attention to the geometry, becomes a matter of effort. It would be wrong, however, to make voluntary attention or the feeling of effort, the *sine qua non* of purposive thinking. Efficient, controlled thought may go on with little or no feeling of effort. Connection after connection may be made, all leading steadily toward the desired end; irrelevant ideas may occur but seldom and, when they do occur, be pushed aside without any struggle. The following account by Galton of his own thinking illustrates this and also the general characteristics of the process of connection in purposive thinking.

"When I am engaged in trying to think anything out, the process of doing so appears to me to be this: The ideas that lie at any moment within my full consciousness seem to attract of their own accord the most appropriate out of a number of other ideas that are lying close at hand, but imperfectly within the range of my consciousness. There seems to be a presence-chamber in my mind where full consciousness holds court, and where two or three ideas are at the same time an audience, and an antechamber full of more or less allied ideas, which is situated just beyond the full ken of consciousness. Out of this antechamber the ideas most nearly allied to those in the presence-chamber appear to be summoned in a mechanically logical way, and to have their turn of audience.

"The successful progress of thought appears to depend—first, on a large attendance in the antechamber; secondly, on the presence there of no ideas except such as are strictly germane to the topic under consideration; thirdly, on the justness of the logical mechanism that issues the summons. The thronging of the antechamber is, I am convinced, altogether beyond my control; if the ideas do not appear, I cannot create them, nor compel them to come. The exclusion of alien ideas is accompanied by a sense of mental effort and volition whenever the topic under consideration is unattractive, otherwise it proceeds automatically, for if an intruding idea finds nothing to cling to, it is unable to hold its place in the antechamber, and slides back again. An animal absorbed in a favorite occupation shows no sign of painful effort of attention; on the contrary, he resents interruption that solicits his attention elsewhere.

"The consequence of all this it that the mind frequently does good work without the slightest exertion."[1]

[1] *Inquiries into Human Faculty*, p. 203.

§ 49. *Reasoning*

The word reasoning has no exact accepted meaning. Its most general meaning, which will be adopted here, is purposive thinking which solves, or tries to solve, new problems. The man who thinks of whipping his horse to make him go out from his barn, does not reason. But the man who, when the horse refuses to go out, procures a bucket of oats, lets the horse begin to eat them and while his attention is thus distracted, gently leads it out through the door, reasons; for he solves a problem for which ordinary habits of thought or action do not suffice. In reasoning, then, we deal with new data or with old data in new ways; we break away from the field of concrete habits and particular associations.

Inductions and Deductions.—The logic books divide reasonings into inductions, in which the examination of many particular facts leads to a general conclusion, and deductions, in which some general conclusion already found leads to another general conclusion or to a judgment about some particular fact. When a student finds that hydrochloric acid and zinc produce hydrogen and chloride, that nitric acid and silver produce certain gases and silver nitrate and so on, and therefore concludes that any acid will combine with any metal to form a salt, he reasons by induction. When he argues that since the sum of the three angles of a triangle equals two right angles, the sum of the two acute angles of a right triangle will equal one right angle, or that the three angles of such and such a particular figure will equal two right angles, he reasons by deduction.

In both cases the process involves the analysis of facts into their elements and the selection of the element that is, or is thought to be, instructive. In the case of the inductive reasoning, the student must have thought, not of the total appearances of the chemicals with which he experimented, but of the elements; acid-quality, metal-quality and salt-quality. In the first case of deductive reasoning, he must have thought, not of the form or direction of the two angles of a right triangle, but of their equality to 'three angles of a triangle minus one right angle.' In the second he discards from attention all the features of the figure (size, shape, etc.) except the 'being a surface inclosed by three straight lines in the same plane.'

The important factors in inductive reasoning are fertility of association, to call up a sufficient number of particular facts; the capacity to select their common ele-

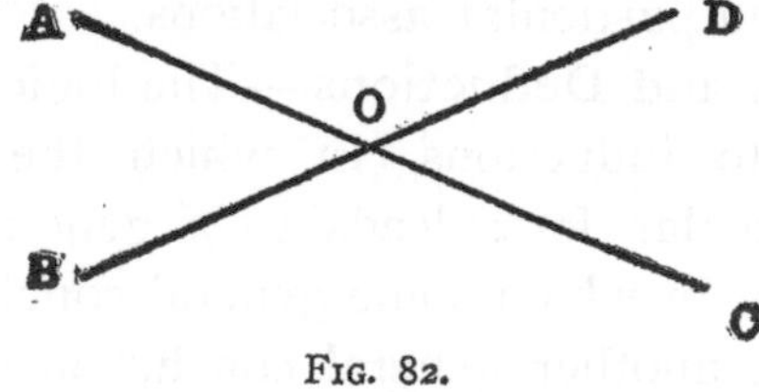

FIG. 82.

ments by the working of the law of dissociation; and the capacity to judge which of the elements is the essential one for the end in view. Fertility of knowledge, power of abstraction and sagacity in selection make the efficient inductive reasoner. One may fail by not having the facts to begin with, by not being able to analyze them or by neglecting their vital feature. Thus one could not reason well about the cause of malaria who had never studied cases of it, or who could not separate the phenomenon as a whole into its conditions, cause, symptoms, effects, and the like; and one could never get the right answer who studied the high body-temperature, or the mental lassitude, or the occurrence in swampy places, neglecting the 'having the malarial parasite in the blood' feature.

The important factors in deductive reasoning are the power of abstraction, enabling one to break up a given fact into its elements, fertility of knowledge of the properties of these elements and sagacity in the choice of the essential one. To take a very simple case, to prove that 'if one straight line cuts another straight line, the vertical angles are equal,' a school-boy must be able to think of the angle A O B (see Fig. 82) as B O D—D O A or as A O C—B O C, and of D O C as A O C—D O A or as B O D—B O C, and of B O D or O A C as a straight line. He must have the sagacity to see that for the end in view he must think of A O B as B O D—D O A in combination with the thought of D O C as A O C—D O A or of A O B as A O C—B O C in combination with the thought of D O C as B O D—B O C.

To take another case, one must, to draw the right conclusion about the treatment of a diseased condition of the throat, be able to distinguish its different symptoms, must attend to the presence of the Klebs-Loeffler bacillus as the vital feature, and know the property of that bacillus as the cause of diphtheria and the property of diphtheria as curable by antitoxin.

We may expect to find efficient reasoning only where the capacities to dissociate and to make associations by partial activity are well developed. Its rarity in comparison with the ability to learn by mere association and to remember, is due to the comparative rarity of these two capacities. When they are present in a high degree and are supported by a wide range of knowledge about the topic in question, the results in reasoning seem to ordinary mortals miraculous. We can hardly keep from believing that the flights of great genius are the result of an inscrutable capacity for being right where others are wrong.

It is, however, possible to understand the miracle,

The purposive thinking of the genius is wonderful, but not because it is of a mysteriously different kind from that of ordinary men. The marvel is in the superior activity of the processes of dissociation or abstraction by which a fact reveals to the genius elements or aspects never before seen in it, and in the superior fertility by which one after another of the consequences of this new insight are passed in review and so used to test its value.

Training in Reasoning.—(1) Facts to reason with are the first essential to progress in reasoning. It is by other facts that the pertinence of any fact is judged; it is by calling up some decisive fact that the selected element brings the thinker nearer to the desired conclusion.

(2) Practice in attending to the parts or elements of facts, in examining each detail, in thinking of things not in their gross total appearance but in their different aspects and with respect to their different features, is the second essential. The student must learn to conquer facts by dividing them.

(3) The greatest aid in this process is comparison. Elements appear in a fact when it is in juxtaposition with others which would never be noticed in it by itself. Thinking things together, putting them in groups, looking for similars and opposites, supplanting the random order of the world's facts by an arrangement into classes,—into likes and unlikes, causes and effects, conditions and dependents and the like,—is the preliminary to insight into the world's nature. It furnishes the opportunity for the law of dissociation to operate.

(4) Practice in criticising one's ideas,—in asking 'Does this fit the problem?' 'Is this a relevant, useful idea?' 'Where will this fact lead?' 'Am I on the right track?'—will improve the power to select wisely and to

resist the attractions of unessential ideas. This process of criticism, of learning to judge whether the idea present is the one essential to the end in view, will be improved (5) by knowledge of the common fallacies or mistakes to which thinking is subject, and of the useful methods of verification of thought by appeal to observation and experiment. Practice in detecting fallacies and verifying conclusions is the business of logic and scientific method, not of psychology.

Exercises

1. Which of the trains of thought of question 3 of the exercises following § 45 seem most purposive or controlled?

2. In which case is it harder to tell whether frequency, recency or intensity is the cause of the connection, in the connections of passage I., of page 251 or in those of passage IV., of page 253?

3. Why?

4. Notice what happens as you try to think of a word meaning 'not capable of being taken away from or given away by the possessor.'

5. Note what happens in your mental life when you think out the answer to the question, 'What are the opposites of because, if, and, adroit, loquacious, to degrade?'

6. Prove the following proposition: The diagonals of a rectangle are equal. Write down every idea you have in the course of thinking out the proof. After you have finished, examine the series of ideas recorded and note instances of selection and of rejection.

7. Compare a passage involving reasoning with a simple descriptive passage of equal length:—[1]

(a) In the number of general notions.
(b) " " " " abstract notions.
(c) " " " " intellectual relationships.
(d) " " " " associations by focal activity.

Experiment 26. Spontaneous and Controlled Association.— Cover the lists of words printed below and look at them only as necessary for the experiment.

[1] Selections of the one sort will be readily found in text books on mathematics, physics, economics and the like; and of the other sort in novels or biographies.

Get a friend to measure, with a stop watch if one is obtainable, the time taken in calling up the things or words suggested by the words in list A. That is, uncover the words at a given signal, looking at the first word. As soon as any thing or word comes to your mind, look at the second; as soon as it arouses an idea look at the third and so on. When the tenth word has called up its associated idea record the time that has elapsed in seeing the ten words and thinking of ten things.

Do the same with lists B, C and D except that the idea called up must mean in every case the opposite of the thing or quality meant by the printed word (*e. g.*, for work you must think *play*, or *be idle* or the like, for friend you must think *enemy* or *foe* or the like).

Compare the times taken in the four cases. Record, so far as you can remember them, any instances of the inhibition of irrelevant or misleading ideas that came to mind in the course of thinking of the opposites of list D.

A.	B.	C.	D.
house	day	permanent	proud
tree	long	to spend	weary
child	boy	to reveal	permit
time	white	motion	genuine
art	outside	separate	to respect
London	good	rude	precise
Napoleon	poor	simple	obnoxious
think	to hate	grand	unitary
red	yes	frequently	scatter
enough	above	broken	particular

Experiment 27. Spontaneous and Controlled Association.—(a) With pencil in hand read the passage that follows, writing in each of the blank spaces the *very first* word that comes to mind as you read. Have some one note the number of seconds which the experiment takes. Read the same passage as before, writing in each of the blank spaces the word which seems to you the right one. Have some one note the time taken as before. Describe the differences between the two mental processes.

The world is too much with us; late and soon,
Getting and spending, we lay waste our powers:
Little we see in Nature that is ——;
We have given our hearts away, a —— boon!

The Sea that bares her bosom to the moon;
The winds that will be —— at all ——;
And are up-gathered now like —— flowers;
For this, for ——, we are out of tune;
It moves us not. Great God! I'd rather be
A —— suckled in a creed ——;
So might I, standing on this —— lea,
Have —— that would make me less ——;
Have sight of Proteus rising from the sea;
Or hear old Triton blow his wreathed horn.

(b) Do likewise with the following passage:—

TRANSPORTATION. — The transporting —— of running water —— as the sixth-power of the velocity. Even at this enormous —— of increase, blocks of stone of many hundreds of tons weight, such as are often found in the —— of glaciers, would require, if carried by ——, an almost incredible ——. But glaciers carry —— resting on their surfaces, and therefore of all sizes, with —— ease. Rock-fragments of thousands of tons —— are —— by them and left in —— path by retreat. Again: fragments carried by water are always more or less bruised, worn, and rounded, while fragments carried on the surface of —— are ——. Again, water-currents set down blocks of stone in —— positions; while glaciers, in their slow melting, often leave them perched in —— positions, and even sometimes as rocking-stones.

References

A. James *Briefer Course,* XVI. (271-279), XXII.
Stout, *Manual,* 447-458.
Titchener, *Outline,* §§ 84-85.

B. James, *Principles,* XXII.

CHAPTER XVIII

The Connections Between Mental States and Acts: Connections of Expression

§ 50. *The General Laws of Human Action*

The same laws which describe the connections between sense stimuli and mental states and between one mental state and another, apply to the connections between mental states and movements.

The Law of Instinct.—Given any mental state, that movement will be made which the inborn constitution of the nervous system has connected with the mental state or part of it. The baby reaches for a bright object seen because by inner organization that sense-presentation connects with that act. For the same reason he puts the object into his mouth when he feels it within his grasp. The boy puts up his arm and wards off a blow, and strikes back at the giver of the blow, because his brain is so organized by nature as to connect those responses with those situations.

The Law of Association.—Given any mental state, that movement will be made which has been connected with it or part of it most frequently, most recently, in the most vivid experience and with the most resulting satisfaction, and which has been so connected with the general system of thought and conduct present. We say five when we think five; we take off our clothes when we decide to go to bed; we shake hands with a caller; we pat a dog; we stroke a kitten; we put a hat on our head and a coat over our shoulders—because in the past we have done so and without discomfort. Each of the factors noted finds illustrations in any day's experiences.

We put cheese in our mouths and keep soap out of our mouths, put our hands in water and not in fire, because the opposite connections have brought discomfort. We say *man* and not *mensch* or *homme* when we mean a man, or sit on chairs rather than on the floor, chiefly because we have made those connections so often. We say, 'How do you do,' to a friend if we see him on the street but do not if we see him in church, because the connection made in the case of the general system has been avoided in the case of the 'in church' system. For the same reason the girl in her 'teens may be of a delicate and ethereal appetite in her 'party system' and in the presence of strangers, but seizes and devours 'pork and beans, and beef and greens' in the 'at home in the pantry' system. Recency is not so common an influence in the case of connections of expression as it is in the case of purely mental connections. Its influence is clearly seen, however, in the experience, common in pronunciation, typewriting and games of skill, of repeating two or three times within a few minutes an error or blunder once made. So also, if you have been signing ten or twelve letters with someone else's name and then turn to a letter of your own, you will often perform the recent act instead of the right and far more frequent one. The influence of vividness or intensity is often hard to separate from that of satisfaction and discomfort, but is witnessed by such facts as the following: In walking up a flight of, say, eight steps which we traverse often in the day time, we always then step out forward instead of up after the eighth step is reached. Yet in walking up them in the dark the situation 'eighth step reached' does not securely produce the movement of stepping out forward, for, though so frequently made, the situation and act have lacked vividness, have been only in the margin of thought and little attended to, since in day-light the vivid and attended-to facts have been the sight of the steps and their surroundings.

The Law of Assimilation in the Case of Connections of Expression.—If the mental state is a new one, that movement will follow it which would follow a familiar state like it. Thus the person unused to the paraphernalia of the breakfast table responds to the sight of a finger bowl by drinking from it; the baby runs to pick up a bird; Sir Walter Raleigh's servant threw a bucket of water on him when he saw him smoking a pipe.

The fact of instinct, the general law of association and its supplement, the law of assimilation, thus are operative in the case of the facts of conduct as well as in the case of those of sense perception and thought.

The Law of Analysis.—The application of the law of dissociation or analysis to movements was made in Chapter XIV. Suffice it to say that elements of complex movements come to appear in isolation when the same movement has been made in many different combinations and that after they acquire thus an independent existence, they enter into new combinations resulting in what are apparently totally new acts. Thus from the complex movements involved in its cries and prattling the infant develops by dissociation the elementary movements involved in articulate speech and gradually combines these elements by association into new words and phrases.

§ 51. *The Will: Spontaneous and Purposive Action.*

Exceptions to the General Law.—No one will deny that nine out of ten or even nine hundred and ninety-nine out of a thousand of human acts occur in accord with these general laws. But do these laws not break down in the case of the few, but real and tremendously significant connections when by an effort of will we supplant the pleasurable by a painful, the frequent by a new, connection? Can man not act against instinct, habit and desire by force of pure will? Such possible exceptions to the common laws of human behavior may best be examined after a distinction between spontaneous and controlled action, similar to the distinction made in the case of thought, has been explained.

Spontaneous and Controlled Action.—Spontaneous, unintentional and involuntary are three synonymous names applied to behavior where the act follows the mental state without any consciousness of purpose, is done without foresight. Controlled, purposive or voluntary action means, on the contrary, behavior in which a purpose is felt, in which we think what we are about and act with foresight. To think, 'I must read that book now,' and to take and open the volume, is a case of voluntary action. When, after I begin to read, my eyes continue to move back and forth across the page, the action is involuntary.

Spontaneous actions may be with or without consciousness. For instance, when one's eyes move in ordinary reading, he may not know whether they move or not, and almost never knows the frequent stops which they make in the course of a line. The name, *Automatic Action*, is used for spontaneous action without consciousness. Purposive action as defined is never unconscious. Spontaneous action is never accompanied by the feeling of effort. Purposive action may or may not be accompanied by the feeling of effort.

Purposive action may occur with or without deliberation. Seeing a pin, picking it up and putting it in the pincushion; taking a sheet of paper on thinking of a letter to be written; going to the door on hearing the sound of the door-bell—are cases of action without deliberation. Seeking a snake and picking it up, if done by one who abhors their slimy writhing but wishes to secure a specimen for a scientific friend; taking a sheet of paper, if done after an argument as to whether one can or cannot afford to order a certain book; walking toward the door as the result of choosing to play rather than work—are cases of action after deliberation.

The feeling of effort is present only in the case of deliberative action and not always then. In deliberative action alternatives are present, from which we select. Whenever the selected alternative is unattractive, is a course of action contrary to natural personal cravings, its acceptance is accompanied by a feeling of effort. Or, conversely, when a rejected alternative is attractive, is a course of action agreeable to natural personal cravings, its inhibition is accompanied by a feeling of effort.

The Nature of the Control.—The control of actions means the control of the mental states leading to them. In no case do we control acts directly, but only by arousing or repressing the feelings which would lead to the acts. In trying to produce an act we try to put ourselves in the frame of mind which will be followed by that act. The struggle to keep from doing a certain thing is the struggle to keep in check or to banish utterly the feelings that will issue in the undesired movements. Of course, of these two processes the former involves also putting out of mind ideas which will prevent the desired act, and the latter keeping in mind ideas which will prevent the undesired act. Thus to produce the act of mailing a letter we try simply to remember 'mail letter, mail letter.' To keep from going to sleep we wash our eyes in cold water to stop their heavy, drooping feeling; we stand up and shake ourselves to banish the relaxation of the muscles; we say to ourselves, 'Go to sleep at this hour with all these tasks undone,—nonsense!', to drive out the willingness to lie back and snooze.

The proper frame of mind necessary to produce an act often implies the feeling of consent, the feeling of 'Yes! Let connections be made. There is no need of further postponement. Go ahead!' Just as in purposive thought, after the contemplation of an idea which has satisfied us with its usefulness as a step in the argument, we may feel a peculiar, 'All right, that will do,' which means that no further deliberation is necessary; so in purposive action, the contemplation of an impulse to action often ends in an 'All right, that will do.' Similarly the proper frame of mind necessary to prevent an act often contains as an important element the *feeling of denial,* the feeling of, 'No! No! Halt connections! Wait!' This also has its counterpart in the control of thought.

In every respect, then, the control of purposive action is the same process as the control of thought. The same selective agency, attention, chooses what thought shall determine action. As in reasoning the sequent thought is not created but only chosen ("if the ideas do not appear, I cannot create them, nor compel them to come"), so in conduct the act is created or 'willed' not directly, but only indirectly through such manipulation of the mental state as will make it the necessary sequent. What is directly selected or rejected in action, as in thought, is a mental state. The only difference is that the associate, the sequent, is in the one case an idea, in the other a movement.

The Real Meaning of Acts of Pure Will.—The facts stated in the preceding paragraphs provide the real meaning and the explanation of those cases where man appears to act contrary to the laws of association, in spite of instinctive tendencies, pleasurable consequences and frequency of connection, by an exertion of pure will. They show first of all that the exertion of pure will influences acts only indirectly by influencing mental states. The will to do a thing is the will to keep a frame of mind that will result in the doing of that thing. "The will is a relation between the mind and *its ideas.*" "The point to which the will is directly applied is always an idea." We do not choose movements, but the ideas leading to movements. In the second place, the contradiction of the laws of association is not real, only apparent. The ascetic who scourges himself really illustrates those very laws, in particular the law of *partial activity;* for his act is the sequent, not of the mere total mental state 'whip in hand,' but of the thought, 'Strike, bruise, crucify your flesh, feel pain for the glory of God! Yes! Yes!', to which his act is the natural sequent. The connection would be unexpected if the instinctive tendencies felt were those of self-preservation, but they are not: they are those of self-sacrifice. It would be unexpected if the painful consequences were attended to, but they are not: the satisfaction of repentance, restitution and peace is the main resultant. It would be unexpected if the antecedent state of mind were that which an ordinary mortal would face when thinking of giving himself a beating, but it is not: the 'Yes! Yes', the feeling of acceptance, means that the ideas that would lead to opposing acts are all banished and that the way is open and unimpeded to the movements of scourging oneself, which are, in view of the circumstances, the most frequent connection. In the third place, since the exertion of pure will works always upon mental states, it is a feature of thought as well as of conduct. Man contributes to the world by knowledge and belief in the same way as by choice and action.

The real fact to which experiences of the choice of the hard instead of the easy and the rare instead of the usual, refer,—the real meaning of the exertion of pure will,—is the law of partial activity,—the power of man to attend to and cherish whatever frame of mind appeals to his general purpose in life or to the ideal of the moment. In rational thinking he may discard the customary and obvious in favor of some abstract element which appeals perhaps to none but him. In controlled action he may banish ordinary likes and dislikes, usual habits and impulses, and elevate to the leadership of his mind some ideal purpose,—some motive which defies the claims of the majority of men and even those of his own past. His will is free in the sense that at any moment what he will attend to and cherish depends upon *him,* upon his attitude toward the situation he confronts. Whether it is free in the further sense that this attitude would be unpredictable even by a perfect intelligence that knew his inborn nature and entire previous experience, is a question unanswered by science and disputed by philosophers.

§ 52. *The Nature of the Mental States Which Precede Movements*

The Problem.—Psychologists have argued much about what kinds of mental states are the antecedents of movements in purposive action. The arguments concern chiefly (1) the so-called *feelings of innervation,* (2) the feeling of *decision,* of *consent,* of *'let this act be,' the fiat,* and (3) the *memory images of the feelings produced by the movement.*

By feelings of innervation are meant feelings directly due to the passage of the nervous impulse to efferent neurones and through them to the muscles. It is very doubtful whether any feelings are so caused. They certainly are not essential to the execution of a purposely made movement. The feeling of decision has been already described. Though of frequent occurrence, notably in action after deliberation, it cannot be regarded as a *sine qua non* of purposive action, as defined in this book; for of the thousand intentional acts of a day, only a small number are preceded by it. The *memory images of the feelings produced by the movement* are of two sorts, *Resident* and *Remote.* By *resident* feelings are meant the feelings of tension, movement and the like *of the moving part,* due to the movement itself. By *remote* feelings are meant the feelings of any sort secondarily caused by the movement, *e.g.,* the sound due to the movements of saying a word, the pressure due to grasping a stick, or the sight of the clinching and clinched fist due to the same movements.

Any Variety of Mental State May Precede a Voluntary Act.—Nearly all writers on psychology seem sure that some special sort of feelings must be present in purposive action. Some think the feeling of decision must always be there; some think that feelings of innervation must be there; nearly all think that at least memory images of the feelings produced by the movement must be there. Only recently has it been argued that after all there is no justification for the assumption that any peculiar sort of feeling is a necessary element of purposive action; that really *any mental state whatever may be the antecedent of an intentional act.* Yet this seems easily demonstrable. For instance, I just now completed the purposive action of writing, 'Yet this seems easily demonstrable.' The act was certain finger and arm movements and certain eye movements involved in guiding them. But my antecedent state of mind contained no images whatever of feelings in my fingers, arms or eyes, nor even of the sight of the words. It was simply the judgment, 'Yet this seems easily demonstrable,' felt with the auditory images of the words. A few hours ago I signed a lease, and I can confidently affirm that the thought antecedent to the act contained no images of any sensations in any way connected with the act of writing my name, but only the auditory images, 'He came to my terms after all.' Professor James, who maintains that "whether or no there be anthing else in the mind at the moment when we consciously will a certain act, a mental conception made up of these sensations (of the movement's results) * * * must be there," (*Principles*, Vol. II, p. 492) gives illustrations which prove precisely that the antecedent to a movement need never have been its *result*. "We say, 'I must go downstairs,' and ere we know it we have risen, walked and turned the handle of a door." (Idem. p. 519) "Hallo! I must lie here no longer," is the antecedent to getting out of bed. (Idem. p. 524).

The Feelings Produced by a Movement Rarely Cause It.—In fact, the doctrine that the image of some one of the previous *results* or *effects* of a movement is its necessary antecedent in purposive action makes the perversest of mistakes. The antecedent is some one of its previous *preliminaries* or *causes*. Occasionally what was first a result or effect of a movement may later be thought of as a preliminary, and so become its antecedent in still later connections, but in general what has *led* to a movement, not what has *come after it*, will lead to it on future occasions. It is not the image of a mouth full of liquid but the sight of the bottle, that makes the baby reach out its hands. It is not the feeling of a brush on one's head, but the thought 'I must comb my hair,' that assists our toilet. It is not the thought of feeling warm but of feeling cold, that commonly makes one build a fire. It is the thought of a bill as due, not as having been paid, which makes us draw a check. We do not move our eyes so as to focus them on an object because we see it clearly, but because we don't. We do not eat because we feel full in imagination, but because we feel empty in reality.

Motives.—So also there is no need of restricting the word motive to any particular class of feelings. Any mental state may serve as a motive. For a motive to an act is simply any fact which assists to be present and to be approved, a mental state which will have the act as its sequent. A motive against the act is simply any fact which hinders the presence and approval of a mental state which will have the act as its sequent. One of the most artificial doctrines about human nature which has ever acquired prominence is the doctrine that pleasure and pain, felt or imagined, are the only motives to action, that a human being is constantly making a conscious or unconscious calculation of the amount of each which the contemplated act will produce, and that his entire behavior is the result of such a lifelong series of complicated sums in addition and substraction. Pleasure and pain do play a leading rôle in determining action, but the cast of characters includes also percepts, ideas and emotions of all sorts.

Exercises

1. State in the case of each of the following whether it is an instinctive or an acquired connection:—

Situation	*Response*
a. A bright light.	Blinking

b.	A bright light.	Pulling down a curtain.
c.	Feeling cold.	Shivering.
d.	Feeling cold.	Opening a radiator.
e.	The sight of a cup of tea.	Drinking it.
f.	The sight of an approaching missile.	Dodging it.
g.	Feeling sleepy.	Closing the eyes.
h.	The thought, 'It is breakfast time'.	Getting up from bed.
i.	The sight of a book.	Opening it at the first page.
j.	Falling.	Clutching at objects.
k.	A blow received.	A blow given.

2. Which three of the following involve many movements acquired through dissociation from more complex movements?—Running, wrestling, singing, playing the piano, climbing, writing.

3. (a) Give two cases of connections of expression acquired chiefly by reason of resulting satisfaction. (b) Two acquired chiefly by reason of resulting discomfort. (c) Two acquired chiefly by reason of mere frequency.

4. Give five instances of connections all ending in the act of shaking hands, the act being in one case spontaneous and unconscious, in the second case spontaneous but conscious, in the third case purposive but without deliberation or effort, in the fourth case purposive and with deliberation but without effort, and in the fifth case with both deliberation and effort.

5. Give five similar instances of connections all ending in the act of saying, 'Yes'.

6. Which part of the following train of thought would probably be operative in arousing action (a) in a gourmand, (b) in a philanthropist, (c) in a proud and honest business man, (d) in a dandy?—"I have only ten dollars. I owe Jones eight. How hungry I am. That woman opposite looks half-starved. Her clothes are as shabby as mine."

7. In a railroad accident a lady was mortally injured. Having but a few hours to live she begged her husband not to leave her. The surgeon called him to help rescue the passengers still confined in the wreck. What will decide which thing the man will do?

8. What statements in § 51 support the following?—"Every act of will requires attention and every concentration of attention is an act of will." (Preyer.)

§ 53. *Suggestion and Imitation*

In General.—To produce a given act in any person implies the arousal in him of the mental state which has that act as its sequent. If the act is the inevitable sequent of the mental state, this is sufficient. To make a baby cry, it is sufficient to make it feel severe pain. To make a man eat, it is sufficient in almost all cases to make him feel very hungry. But usually the act will only follow the mental state on condition that the latter is without opposition, is attended to exclusively, is freed from the influence of conflicting ideas. To produce a given act in any person thus commonly implies the arousal of the mental state which has that act as its sequent and also the suppression of conflicting or competing mental states.

Conflicting ideas may be (1) prevented from appearing at all or (2) inhibited in the course of deliberation. They may be inhibited by motives in the shape of promises, arguments, entreaties, threats and the like which weaken them or which strengthen contrary ideas.

Suggestion.—There will therefore be two methods of arousing an act: (1) by *Suggestion* and (2) by *Persuasion.* In cases of suggestion, the idea which tends to result in the act is so aroused in the mind that few or no conflicting ideas will appear; the person is prevented so far as possible from deliberating, in the hope that the mere tendency of the idea itself to work out into the act will suffice. In cases of persuasion, the idea which tends to result in the act is so aroused in the mind that it will possess motives to support it even at the cost of the arousal of conflicting ideas as well; the person is encouraged to deliberate and to consider the motives in the hope that those favoring the act will prevail.

The power of suggestion depends upon the fact that any idea does tend to result in its appropriate act if no competing idea or physical impediment prevents it. Suggestion as a method of control is especially useful (1) in cases where the individual *could* not rightly value the motives, and (2) in cases where it is important that the individual should do the right thing, but is relatively unimportant that he should learn to rightly value the motives. Thus to argue with a homicidal maniac would be folly, and to attempt to teach a three-year-old child why he should not cry, would be a waste of time. It is much better to say to the maniac who approaches with drawn knife, 'You have forgotten your spectacles,' and to the crying baby, 'Now you are really one of the bravest boys, I know. Just a minute and you won't cry any more. I know you didn't mean to. You are all right now.' Suggestion as a method of control is risky in cases where training in judgment and choice is one chief benefit of the act. It is bad for any rational being to be forever hoodwinked into doing this, that and the other.

Differences in the degree of suggestibility,—in the tendency to accept ideas and neglect conflicting ideas,—are important amongst individual differences. Some people live continually in a state approaching that of a hypnotized person. They do and believe whatever they are told; they never make a logical decision; they are the prey of the last person who sees them. At the other extreme is the stolid but hard-headed type that figures everything out, that greets the most adroit suggestion with a, 'Huh! So you want me to do something. Well! I'll think it over.' When only half awake, when asleep, and above all in the hypnotic and certain other trance states we all lapse into a more and more suggestible condition.

Imitation.—The word imitation is now used in psychology to mean two different facts. The first is the general fact of the repetition of one man's thoughts and acts by other men. In this sense imitation means the opposite of invention, and includes perhaps ninety-nine per cent. of life; for a really new thing in thought or conduct is extremely rare. The second meaning is the fact of the influence of the concrete behavior of one individual upon other individuals, as opposed to the influence of explanations, commands, lessons and the like. In this narrower sense imitation means the influence of personal example. It is imitation in this second sense that will be discussed here.

Among the most numerous and the most important causes of the ideas producing action in a human being are the acts of other human beings. Manners, accent, the usages of language, style in dress and appearance,—in a word, the minor phases of human behavior,—are guided almost exclusively by them. They also control the morals, business habits and political action of many men on many occasions. As the physical environment decides in large measure what things a man shall see and hear, so the social environment decides in large measure what he shall do and feel.

The acts of other people exert a twofold influence: (1) that of stimuli to action and (2) that of models by which the satisfactoriness of an act is judged. Thus (1) A's going to school may arouse in B the idea and act of going to school, or (2) A's style of speech may be B's model, to speak as A does giving him satisfaction and so being the goal of his trials. As stimuli to action other people's acts are as a rule more potent than explanations, precepts and advice because they are clear and concrete. It is, for instance, easy to *show* a servant how to turn on and off the electric light in a room, but very hard to *tell* him how. They also have strong suggestive force, since to see other people doing a thing inhibits any ideas of the act's impossibility or undesirability. If everyone else is rushing down the street, the idea of so doing tends to be deprived of opposition.

As models by which to judge one's own acts, the acts of other people have the advantage over abstract principles or verbal descriptions, of being far more clear and vivid. No explanation of the essentials of a graceful gesture can in these respects equal the actual sight of it as made by the teacher. The student of music can compare the tone he produces with that actually produced by his master far better than with an ideal constructed from general statements.

Exercises

1. What statements in § 53 support the following?—

"What we do, when we want to pursue any line of conduct, is to hold that action clearly in mind and dismiss all impeding or inhibiting thoughts. When we want to influence any one to do a particular thing, we try so to present it to him that it completely fills his mind. We try to get him to think of the action without thinking of any contradictory action. If we want him to go West, we can accomplish the result if we can get him to think of going West without having the ideas of going East or of standing still arise in his mind and check action. If you can get him to think of going to Kansas City over the Chicago & Alton, he will go to Kansas City over the Chicago & Alton, and nothing but a competing idea or physical impediment can stop him. If he is so taken up with the idea of Chicago & Alton that the name of no other means of transportation enters his mind, and if he is so situated that no physical impediment (sickness, lack of money, etc.) hinders him, he will start at once to go to the destination thought of and over the route thought of. All we can do is to get the thought into the mind and in an automatic manner the thought will suggest the action." (Scott, *Theory of Advertising*, pp. 51-52.)

2. Read Mark Antony's speech over Caesar's body (*Julius Caesar*, Act III., Scene II., *passim*). Note three or four parts

which make prominent use of suggestion and three or four parts which make prominent use of persuasion.

3. Why do political parties spend money in printing such apparently unconvincing stuff as, 'Vote Under the Eagle', or 'Vote the Straight Democratic Ticket?'

4. Collect from magazines four advertisements that depend for success chiefly upon suggestion. Four that depend chiefly on persuasion.

5. What risk is run by the parent or teacher who in educating children relies upon suggestion and imitation rather than argument and principles?

§ 54. *Individual Differences in the Life of Action*

Their Amount.—Individuals differ by inborn constitution with respect to the intensity of certain desires and interests, the capacities for connecting acts with mental states speedily, surely and permanently, the capacities for attending to abstract considerations, the capacities for resisting the strain of effort, and the other factors which influence human action. They differ by training in the kinds of mental states which they feel, in the elements of these to which they attend, in the acts which are connected therewith and in the ways in which the inborn instincts and capacities just mentioned are modified. There is perhaps no desire so universal as not to be absent in some human being and no connection between mental state and act so absurd and unlikely as not to have somewhere existed. I dare say that the thought of four times seven may have made some maniac jump with glee, and impelled some other to cut his throat. The differences in inborn desires and interests and tendencies to action will, in general, be less than the differences in inborn capacities to connect and attend, and these will, in general, be less than the differences in acquired ideas and habits.

Little is known of the amounts of difference in these various respects or of the types or species of character into which human beings may perhaps be divided. Anyone may at least be sure that it is unsafe to prophesy the behavior of anyone else on the basis of what he himself would do and that it is unjust to judge the behavior of anyone else on the basis of the motives which he himself would have felt. The following differences and types, by no means exactly duplicated in reality, are worthy of study as samples of present incomplete knowledge of individual differences in controlled action:—

Differences in the Antecedents of Action.—Individuals may be ranked in a series according to the extent to which abstract ideas serve as the antecedents of action. At one extreme are those men and women who, like the lower animals, react only to some concrete particular situation. They live by special habits, not by general rules. They can work for a man, but not for a cause. They can fight a fire or a seen enemy, but not a principle like falsity or injustice. They can worship an idol or a saint, but not truth or righteousness. At the other extreme are those who can break up a total fact into its elements and react to one quality whenever found, to injustice whether experienced from friend or enemy, to truth whether found in their creed or another's. Such men and women progress from special habits to general principles of behavior, originate customs and modify social codes. They include the geniuses of action, and also its fanatics. Most men and women occupy stations near the middle of such a scale. They act in the main in response to concrete facts, but possess a few general practices, avoiding 'crime,' refusing to be 'unladylike,' and doing 'their duty,' when an act possesses sufficiently obviously the abstract quality in question.

The Impulsive Type.—Individuals may also be ranked in a series according to the strength of the tendency of a mental state to call up action compared with its tendency to call up another mental state. At one extreme is the man or woman who can hardly have any idea without following it by its connected act. 'John is in town; let's go and see John,' and he seizes his hat. 'Where is my hat?', and she runs about in search for it. At the other extreme is the one who can rarely get so far as to *do* anything about anything. 'John is in town. I wonder where he lives. Would he be at home now if we should call? Perhaps he won't want visitors yet. It's a disagreeable day anyway. He rather likes company, though. It would take all the evening. I'm not sure what I'd best do,' and so on. 'Where is my hat? I probably may not find it if I look for it. It will do no harm to go out bare-headed. Still it would look queer. I wonder if it is in that closet. Perhaps I'd better look. Still I feel sure I had it in this room. Where shall I look for it?', and so on for twice the time it would take to ransack the house. The first extreme we may call the *Impulsive,* the latter the reflective, or, still better, since reflective is commonly used of necessary thoughtfulness, the *Pondering,* individual. As before, most of us occupy a station midway between the extremes. The terms (A) *Explosive Will* and (B) *Obstructed Will,* have been used by Professor James, and others following him, to refer to these extreme types and also in general to (A) individuals who act too much, too quickly and in the wrong direction because impulses are too strong and inhibition too weak, and to (B) individuals who act too little, too late and in the wrong direction because impulses are too weak and inhibitions too strong.

§ 55. *The Control of the Life of Action*

The good and efficient character implies the subjugation of those instinctive tendencies to action which injure oneself or others, the energetic action of desirable ones, the presence of worthy ideals and the connection of these with appropriate acts, a multiplicity of useful habits, the power to see and react to the element of a situation which will issue in an act producing the best results, the power to react to barren abstractions such as *ought, right* and *true,* the power to delay decision until enough evidence is in to warrant one in deciding, the power to refrain from delaying it too long, and the power to stand the strain of effort implied in choosing a relatively unattractive course of behavior.

The Elements of Moral Training.—The training of character is correspondingly complex. Useful instincts must be given a chance to exercise themselves and become habits. Harmful instinctive responses must be inhibited through lack of stimulus, through the substitution of desirable ones or through actual resultant discomfort, as best fits each special case. The mind must be supplied with noble ideas through the right examples at home, in school, in the world at large and in books. These ideas must be made to issue in appropriate action or they may be worse than useless. The capacity to examine any situation and see what the essential fact in it which should decide action is, must be constantly exercised and guided. The habits of letting 'It is right' or 'It is best' or 'It will be for the real welfare of the world' or the like, be an absolutely final warrant for action must be firmly fixed. The will must be prevented alike from precipitate responses and from dawdling indecision. The power to banish from mind attractive but unworthy ideas, and to go on one's way regardless of the effort involved in so doing, must be gradually built up. Especially important is the actual formation of definite habits. If a man does what is useful and right he will soon gain proper ideas of social efficiency and of morals. If he learns to do the right thing in a thousand particular situations, he will, so far as he has the capacity, gain the power to see what act a new situation demands. If he is made to obey a thousand particular, 'This is right's and 'That is right's, he will, so far as he has the capacity, come to connect respect and obedience with the abstractly right and true. If he does what he has to do well and treats his fellow beings as he should in the thousands of situations of the ordinary course of life, he will gain the power to conquer attractive counter-impulses.

Common Mistakes in Moral Training.—The commonest error is to expect people to become efficient and decent by some mysterious influences from lessons or sermons or good resolutions or what not. We forget that character means the connections between mental states and acts, and that the only way to have connections is to make them. Men become efficient and decent only by behaving efficiently and decently. To work is the only cure for laziness; to give is the only cure for stinginess; to tell the truth is the only cure for lying.

There are many more blunders in our dealings with ourselves and other men from which knowledge of the psychology of human action should rescue us. Of these, two or three are so common as to deserve special mention:—

(1) *To fail to foster the desirable instincts.* Babies are rarely given much attention except when their parents are annoyed by them or wish to pet and display them. They get nothing but neglect for playing quietly, but are

fondled and bribed when they become sufficiently obnoxious. When by chance they behave modestly and obediently, they are unnoticed; but their early efforts at impertinence, self-will and vanity arouse amusement and comment. By the time the two-year-old baby has become a ten-year-old boy the result is often intolerable, and the father who laughed at the infantile self-will is amazed to find an ill-mannered, selfish, petulant son. He then makes an equal error, expecting (2) *to inhibit directly by resulting discomfort a fully formed habit.* He scolds and punishes the boy for the acts he encouraged in the baby. He may mend the boy's manners, but he loses his confidence. He may prevent certain acts for the time being, but they will probably recur when the boy becomes old enough to fear punishment no longer, or when circumstances are such that the act will not be discovered.

(3) *To value the feeling of effort for its own sake.* The feeling of effort is found in efficient and good men; it is a frequent accompaniment of great and noble deeds. As a result we tend to think of it as itself a desirable thing, and to use its presence as a test of the value of any act. 'This is hard; therefore it is right. I do not wish to do this; therefore I ought,' was a common enough reasoning of our Puritan ancestors. '*You* do not wish to do this; therefore *you* ought,' was still commoner. And to-day many a one does, and makes others do, useless acts because they are hard and because their doing will test and increase the power to stand the strain of effort. This is doubly a mistake. The chance to improve character by the performance of concretely useful acts, productive of concretely useful habits, is wasted; and the one who makes the effort, stands the strain, is being taught the lesson that, though he does stand the strain,

nothing comes of it, unless perhaps this power of concentration about which his master disclaims. There are enough useful acts to be done to give all the training in self-control that anyone could ask, and these will increase self-control far more surely, for they will demonstrate that it is worth while.

(4) *To regard quantity of action as a sign of energy.* It is an American fashion to regard repose as indolence and 'hustle' as accomplishment. But in reality a vast amount of action may come from a small amount of energy, when none is expended for inhibition and control. In well-directed action far more energy is consumed in restraining and guiding conduct than in merely arousing it. Indeed, over-action is a recognized symptom of nervous weakness. Men learn efficiency in action by learning to omit erroneous acts and to keep all acts under rigid control. Not quantity, but balance,—the preservation of the golden mean in action,—is the best symptom of energy or strength.

Exercises

1. Illustrate from your own acquaintance or from fiction, extreme inability to act on abstract and general ideas.
2. Illustrate similarly a predominant tendency for ideas to call up other ideas rather than acts.
3. Illustrate similarly an explosive will due to excessive impulsion.
4. Illustrate similarly an explosive will due to a lack of inhibition.
5. Illustrate similarly an obstructed will due to excessive inhibition.
6. Illustrate similarly an obstructed will due to a lack of impulsion.
7. What did Dr. Clouston probably mean by this statement: "You Americans wear too much expression on your faces ...... The duller countenances of the British population be-

token a better scheme of life." (Quoted by James in his *Talks to Teachers on Psychology,* p. 208.)

References

A. James, *Briefer Course,* XXVI.
Stout, *Manual,* 581-616.
Titchener, *Outline,* §§ 62-69.
Angell, *Psychology,* XX., XXI., XXII.
B. Ebbinghaus, *Grundzüge,* §§ 68-69.
James, *Principles,* XXVI.
Wundt, *Physiologische Pyschologie,* XVII.

References on Imitation and Suggestion

Stout, *Manual,* 269-275.
James, *Principles,* XXVII.
Wundt, *Physiologische Psychologie,* XX (§ 3).

CHAPTER XIX

Movements

§ 56. *Acts of Skill*

So far the connections of mental states with bodily movements have been treated broadly and from the point of view of the general conduct of life. From this point of view the exact nature of the movement is of little consequence, the main issue being whether or not a movement of a certain general character shall or shall not be made. In the case of what are called acts of skill the same general problem appears, but the main issue is now: Just what movement shall be made; just how extensive or energetic or long in duration shall it be? Life as a whole is made up of both such movements as are made in playing chess, where *what you do* counts, and of such movements as are made in billiards or lawn tennis, where the thing of importance is *how you do it.* The question before was: 'Given any mental state, what thing shall be done?' The question now is: 'What causes a certain definite, precise movement or series of movements?'

The Acquisition of Skill.—The same law of association operates here as elsewhere. A single illustration will suffice. In drawing a straight line, the situation is the sight of the paper, the feeling of the pencil and of one's arm and fingers in position, and the command or idea that is connected with the act of drawing a straight line. As the movement is made new sensations arise from the sight of so much of the line as has been already drawn, from the movements already made and from the new position taken; the continuation of the movement is the sequent of these as well as of the original mental state; and so on until the movement is complete, each successive part of the movement furnishing new sensations which, arousing their appropriate connections, modify the further course of the movement. Let the reader draw rapidly a line between the two lines of Fig. 83

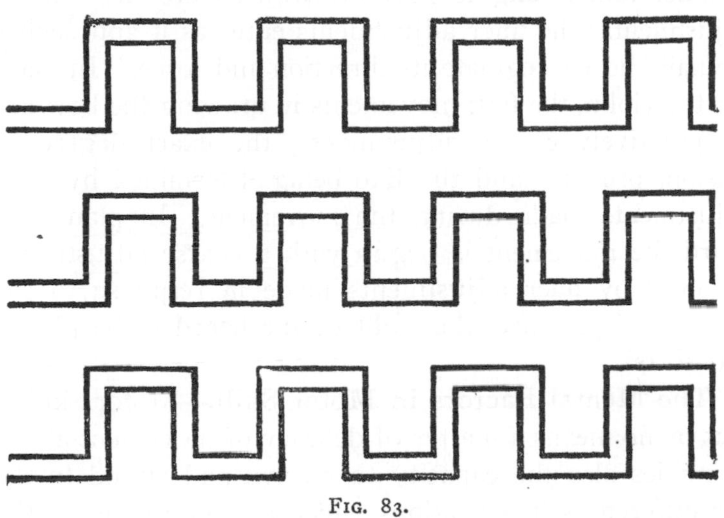

FIG. 83.

without touching either and he will realize this process of continual arousal of alterations in the movement by new sensations produced by it. When you see the pencil going too far down toward one line, you alter its direction; when you have made one or two touches, you decrease the speed. Just how you initiate, guide and alter your movement will depend upon what inborn capacity for steadiness and precision of movement you possess and what previous practice you have had; *i.e.*, upon what connections have been made between this and that guiding sensation and this or that alteration of the movement.

Motor Skill means the existence of certain connections whereby the guiding sensations arouse appropriate movements. *Practice* means the formation of such connections. A skilled movement may commonly be divided into the *coarser* adjustments with which it starts and the *finer* adjustments which come into play in response to the guiding sensations. Thus, in driving a nail, lifting the hammer and letting it start downwards are the coarser adjustments; the finer adjustments enter as it approaches the nail and we regulate its direction and force. In playing the violin, the first movements in drawing the bow are comparatively coarse adjustments, the exact degree of tension, pressure and the like being determined by finer adjustments made during the movement. In planing a board the movement is begun with a coarse adjustment, followed by finer adjustments made in response to the feelings of pressure, the sight of the board to be planed and so on.

The Mental Factors in Motor Skill.—Motor skill is thus by no means a matter of delicacy of movement alone. It implies also the capacity to receive and attend to the fine differences in sensations which are the guides to the finer adjustments, and, most important of all, the capacity to make connections between sensations and movements, to eliminate the unnecessary and undesirable movements. These capacities improve with maturity, and with training, provided the successful connections are rewarded by resultant satisfaction. As a general rule the capacities for the coarser adjustments mature earlier in life than those for the finer adjustments.

Skill in movements is by no means primarily a matter of the arms and hands. The movements of the vocal chords in speech and singing and of the eyes in bringing objects into clearest vision are among the most delicately adjusted movements made by man. In most handicrafts the eyes co-operate in the movements as well as furnish guiding sensations. The movements of the facial muscles by which interest, amusement, enthusiasm and the like are expressed, are often extremely delicate and in the case of actors may be the result of long continued practice.

Skill is improved by (1) deliberately following certain rules which can be learned by mere thought, and (2) by unconsciously dropping inefficient and emphasizing efficient connections in the course of practice. The first factor, the learning by explanations, may be called the acquisition of *Form;* the second factor, the learning by trial and error, or better by the selection of chance successes, may be called the acquisition of *Execution.* The golf player may learn outright what is the right way to hit the ball, how and where to stand, how to hold the club, and the like. This is learning *form.* But the actual associations between the sight of the ball and the exact movements necessary to drive it a hundred and sixty yards, must be patiently built up by the 'try, try again' method.

Exercises

Experiment 28. The Acquisition of Skill.—Make some new combination of movements; *e. g.,* that of drawing a circle with one hand while drawing a straight line with the other. Repeat the process until a fair degree of skill is secured. Notice the tendency for the two hands to move in accord and the difficulty at the start of inhibiting undesirable movements. Note any instances of movements hard to avoid because of their frequent connection with similar situations in the past.

Experiment 29. The Influence of Practice on Motor Skill.—Procure some book or magazine which you are free to mark or destroy. Select 50 pages, in each of which the space between lines of print is the same. Cut them so as to leave 21 lines on each page. Have ready a sharp pencil, and a watch with a second hand. At a fixed time, say when the minute hand is at 14 and the second hand at 60, begin to draw a line between every two lines of print as fast as you can without touching the print in any place. Draw first between the first and second lines from left to right, then around the right end of the second line and back between the second and third lines from right to left and so on until 20 lines have been drawn. Note and record the time of completion and so obtain the number of seconds taken to make the movements.

Make in all 30 or more 20-line tests. Do not make more than 5 or 6 at a time. Try to keep the number of touches at zero and to reduce the time to as low a figure as possible. Compare the first 4 with the last 4 records with respect to time (and touches, if any were made). Compare the first, second, third and last quarters of the total series. Make as clear and complete a statement as you can of the effect of the practice.

If this experiment were to be used as a means of measuring the influence of practice with certainty and precision, what precautions should be taken with respect to avoiding the influence of unfair physical conditions (*e. g.*, light), fatigue, variations in interest and attention and other disturbing factors?

§ 57. *The Connections between Sense Stimuli and Movements*

Automatic Connections.—If the order of our chapters were the order of the development of mental life, the connections between physical stimulations of the sense organs and bodily movements would have been the first group of connections described. Physical stimuli connect with movements earlier in life than they connect with sense impressions and long before sense impressions connect with other mental states.

The order is in fact:—

(1) Connections of physical stimuli with movements.

(2) Connections of physical stimuli with sense impressions, emotions and other feelings of the first intention.

(3) Connections of sense impressions with movements.

(4) Connections of one mental state with another and of mental states of the second and third intentions with movement.

The early connections between stimulus and movement are all unlearned or instinctive. The increased heart-beat in response to physical activity, the primitive embryonic movements, the reaction of the pupil to light and the like are samples of the provision by nature of responses to stimuli which are not even felt. Many such connections persist. Processes go on in the body in response to external and internal stimuli which are not dreamt of in the philosophy of conscious life.

There is a second group of such connections which come much later in life and represent the relics of processes which originally involved physical stimulus, feelings of the first intention and bodily movement. By continued use such connections come to drop the middle term. For instance, walking involves, at first, sensations of sight, pressure, position and motion, which connect with the appropriate movements of the legs and balancing muscles; but in adult life we walk along absorbed in conversation or thought with apparently no such sensations. I say 'apparently' because it is conceivable that the feelings are there but so little attended to as to pass unnoticed. At all events they are so little in evidence that for practical purposes they may be considered absent.

When the physical stimulus arouses a movement *directly* instead of *via some feeling,* the response is called an *Automatic Movement* or an *Automatic Act*, and a series of such connections is called automatic conduct or automatic behavior or automatic action. *Instinctive automatic behavior* is probably common in the very low forms of animal life, such as the protozoa, and in human life before, and perhaps for some weeks after, birth. It persists in many of the fundamental physiological activities. *Acquired automatic behavior* represents nature's economy in leaving unattended to, and even unfelt, those stimuli to which we have gained a perfect habit of response. Just as the thought of 2 times 8 produces the thought of 16 without the reappearance of the long process of learning which was originally necessary, so the touch of the pavement produces the act of walking without perhaps any feeling whatever.

There are all degrees of weakening of the mental state in habitual connections, from the connection so firmly fixed that no sensation can be discerned, up to the connection in which attention is just beginning to be somewhat freed from thinking one by one of the sensations which guide the movement. In learning to play a piece on the piano, to ride a bicycle or to knit, one gradually passes from full consciousness of what one sees and hears and does to such an almost complete absence of feelings concerned with the act that one can think of something else at the time with no effort whatever.

The Function of Automatic Connections.—The saving of time due to this release of attention, and, perhaps, of all feeling, from fully formed habits, is enormous. In so far as the movements of the eyes in reading become automatic, attention can be devoted to the meaning of the words read; in so far as the movements necessary to feed oneself become automatic, the newspaper can be devoured with the breakfast. If the operations of dressing, eating, walking, reading, sewing and the like were all accompanied by the attentive consciousness which went with them in their early appearances, half our days would be spent in getting them done. It is necessary for the efficiency of mental life that many habits should be made thus self-controlling, should be practiced until they make no demands upon mental life proper. Indeed in general we think about things so as eventually to do them without thought. It should be the fate of every connection to progress toward automatic behavior. It is extravagant to waste attention on minor connections which do not deserve it. A student who was forced by circumstances to spend much time in the society of some stupid people, found that by making automatic the habit of responding to a certain general tone by 'Exactly' or 'Certainly,' to another tone by 'Indeed!' or 'Well! Well!' and to still another by, 'Your own judgment on that question would be better than mine,' she could carry on her own meditations almost as well as if by herself. One reason perhaps for the absent-mindedness of gifted men is that they have learned to leave all the small matters of life to take care of themselves and so occasionally blunder by making an automatic response at an improper time. It is better to occasionally enter a neighbor's house, or try to light the gas with a pencil or greet your wife on the street with a pleasant 'And how is your husband's health?', than to think all day long about trifles.

Exercises

1. Name six instinctive automatic connections.

2. What name is given in § 4 to the instinctive automatic connections?

3. Observe by looking in a glass what happens to the pupils of your eyes when you come into a bright room after eight or ten minutes in a very dark room. Would you know what happened to them from direct feeling alone?

4. Name six acquired connections which you make automatically or nearly so.

5. The conjurer Houdin is reported to have been able to keep four balls in the air quite automatically, in fact to do so

while steadily reading a book. Give similar instances showing the degree of complexity possible in automatic connections.

6. Which would be harder, to learn to walk and sew at the same time or to read and sew at the same time?

7. Why is to learn to talk and sew at the same time easier than either?

§ 58. *Movements as Antecedents*

Movements, though they do not directly arouse, do indirectly react on mental states. Any movement serves as a stimulus to the sense organs,—of the eye, if it is seen; of the skin, if it causes tension or folding; of the joints, if a bone is moved; of the muscle itself in any case. Every turn of the eyes, every change of facial expression, every contraction of the vocal chords, every posture of the body, every extension of flexion of a finger, thus plays a part in determining the course of the stream of thought. Just as a multitude of sights and sounds sets at work the forces of sensation and produces new mental states, so the multiplicity of bodily movements produces a crop of secondarily caused sensations, which feature in later thought.

Just what and how great a part movements play as stimuli to sensations, is not known. But it is surely not unimportant. The images of words in which thought is carried on are often motor images of the movements made in speech. The feelings of strain, irritation and perplexity, are very probably due to conditions of general muscle tension. One theory of the fusion of sensations into percepts is that we feel as one thing whatever combination of sensations is responded to by a single movement or a connected series of movements. Some thinkers assert that without bodily movement, controlled thought cannot even take place. The feeling of self or personality, which is one element of almost all mental states, is in large measure due to the ever present stimuli from the muscular tension of the body, the unnoticed movements of breathing, and the like. The feelings of the distances of objects arise in part from feelings of the movements of the eyes made in converging for near and diverging for far objects. General satisfaction and dissatisfaction are, by one theory, explained as the feelings caused by movements of extension or approach and of flexion or withdrawal respectively.

From these and similar facts and theories, it is certain that the indirect contribution of movements to thoughts and feelings is a large one, and one upon which man relies for the material for some of his most important judgments.

Exercises

1. Which looks longer in Fig. 84, the vertical or the horizontal line? Measure the lines. What fact, in addition to the fact that it is harder to move the eyes in a vertical than a horizontal direction, is needed to explain the appearance?

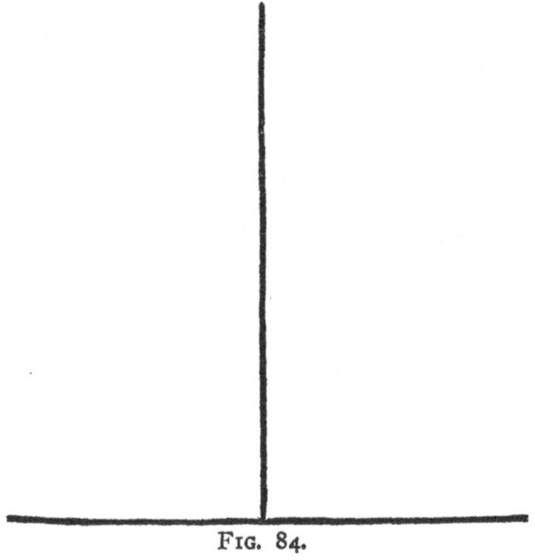

Fig. 84.

2. Can you discover in yourself feelings due to movements of the sort described in the following passages?—

"In consenting and negating, and in making a mental effort, the movements seem more complex, and I find them harder to describe. The opening and closing of the glottis play a great part in these operations, and, less distinctly, the movements of the soft palate, etc., shutting off the posterior nares from the mouth. My glottis is like a sensitive valve, intercepting my breath instantaneously at every mental hesitation or felt aversion to the objects of my thought, and as quickly opening, to let the air pass through my throat and nose, the moment the repugnance is overcome. The feeling of the movement of this air is, in me, one strong ingredient of the feeling of assent. The movements of the muscles of the brow and eyelids also respond very sensitively to every fluctuation in the agreeableness or disagreeableness of what comes before my mind.

In *effort* of any sort, contractions of the jaw-muscles and of those of respiration are added to those of the brow and glottis, and thus the feeling passes out of the head properly so called." James, *Principles,* I., 301.

Experiment 30. Movements as Stimuli to Mental States.—Lie down and let all your muscles relax until you are perfectly limp and easy and without any tension anywhere. Let the muscles of the face relax as well as those of the rest of the body. Rest thus for ten minutes or more. Then jump up, frown, set your teeth, clinch your fists and stalk back and forth with quick, vigorous and jerky movements. How did you feel in the two cases?

References

A. James, *Briefer Course,* XXIII., X.
Stout, *Manual,* 99-102.

B. Ebbinghaus, *Grundzüge,* § 65.
James, *Principles,* XXIII., IV.
Wundt, *Physiologische Psychologie* XIV., § 3.

CHAPTER XX

Selective Processes

§ 59. *Attention and Neglect*

Attention.—In the last seven chapters are frequent references to the facts of attention, the fact (1) that of any mental state some one portion is predominant,—is more likely than others to be operative in causing the sequent mental state or act; and the fact (2) that of many feelings felt, only a few are noticed, dwelt upon, allowed to play leading parts in influencing the future course of thought and action. Chapter VII contained a brief description of the facts of attention. It is now necessary to study their causation; to answer the questions: 'What determines which part of a mental state will be focal? Which mental states will be selected, dwelt upon, allowed to weigh heavily in mental life and conduct?'

Here as elsewhere (1) original nature, (2) the influence of experience and (3) accidental causes share in producing the result. What will be felt as clear, emphatic and focal, what will be selected and dwelt upon, what in short will be attended to, by any individual, will be that mental state or that feature of a mental state which is attractive because of (1) the original tendencies to attend with which nature endows us, because of (2) the habits of attention which have been found by the individual in question to be desirable or because of (3) some accidental cause. The original tendencies to attend may be called instinctive interests; the acquired tendencies to attend may be called acquired interests.

Instinctive Attention.—Some of the more important instinctive tendencies are to attend, other things being equal to:—

(1) Moving objects rather than still objects.
(2) Other human beings and living animals rather than plants or inanimate objects.
(3) Clear rather than obscure or indefinite objects.
(4) Intense rather than weak stimuli.
(5) Novel rather than familiar objects (unless the latter have special advantages).
(6) Pleasurable rather than painful stimuli.
(7) Expected rather than unexpected stimuli.

These tendencies are fairly common to all human beings, though individual differences exist with respect to the amount of strength of each.

Like instincts in general, these instinctive interests may be delayed. Obvious illustrations are the interest in living animals and the interest in the opposite sex. Little is known of the exact time of maturing of instinctive tendencies to attend, because in actual life the influence of original nature is often inextricably conjoined with that of experience. No one can yet say, for instance, how far the tendency to attend to the number aspect of any stimulus,—to count objects,—is a delayed instinct and how far it is an acquired habit.

Acquired Attention—In habits of attention there is amongst individuals a tremendous diversity due to the moderate differences in the instinctive tendencies from which the habits develop, the greater differences in capacities, and the still greater differences in the experiences which life affords to different individuals. We all come to attend in general to spoken words more than to coughs, laughs, sneezes and the like; to facial expression more than to movements of the chest; to the weather more than to the character of the soil. In these cases experience teaches all much the same lessons. But on the whole each individual acquires interests in a special circle of friends, special divisions of knowledge, a special profession or trade, a special locality, and so with the many objects of modern civilized life.

The forces in forming habits of attention, and in deciding what thing or feature out of several will in any given situation be attended to, are the frequency, recency and intensity of attention to the thing on previous occasions, resultant pleasure, and harmony with the general set of the mind. Of these, resultant pleasure is by far the most important. Mere frequency and recency of attention will in fact produce inattention or disregard if the consequences are unsatisfactory or even indifferent; for frequency breeds familiarity and monotony and by original nature the familiar and monotonous is disregarded in favor of the novel. In the long run attention is more and more given to those things attention to which produces felt satisfaction.

Voluntary Attention.—So-called voluntary attention,—*i.e.*, attending with effort and deliberately neglecting the thing which appeals to instinctive interests or pleasurable habits of attention,—seems unexplainable by the laws of instinct and association. Why, for instance, does a boy attend with effort to the words of his spelling lesson when the sound of a band and the vision through the window of a circus parade invite him? As a matter of fact he usually does not. When he does, it is because some idea or feeling in connection with the situation makes the attending to the spelling words more satisfactory to him than attending to the parade. In and of themselves the spelling words would speedily give way to the parade. But the situation is: 'spelling words to look at and think of—please father—show my grit—I'm weak if I don't do it—of course they must be learned first, and the like,' and if these ideals of duty and achievement are highly enough esteemed, the spelling words are clothed with an attractiveness derived from remote aims and enjoyments which is stronger and wins. It is not that the unsatisfying conquers the desirable; but that what is undesirable in itself may be so suffused by the desirability of its connections as to seem the more desirable to the total frame of mind. It is not that men attend, some only to the attractive and others, of a firmer fibre, to the repugnant. The real difference is that some feel satisfaction only in the directly pleasurable, the selfish rewards, the narrow and immediate outcome; whereas others feel satisfaction in the prospects of far off benefits, in the welfare of others, and in the general and eventual outcome which their entire system of ideas and purposes holds in view. The thing to be accounted for is not a difference in the laws of attention but a difference in taste or preference. Whether the proverbial, 'There is no accounting for tastes' be true or not will be seen in a later section. The fact of moment here is the fortunate one that men may have a preference for the eventually useful, the abstractly good and the eternally right as well as for beer and skittles.

The case of voluntary attention, attention against resistance, is one case of the general fact of derived attention. Any thing may gain attention not only from its intrinsic qualities (immediate attention), but also from its associations. Derived attention may or may not imply effort, may minister to higher or lower impulses. Attention to a dollar bill is derived but commonly implies no feeling of effort. Fagin's attention to Oliver Twist, derived from the idea of making him a thief, was of course in the service of a distinctly low motive.

One more fact of the development of tendencies to attend deserves notice,—namely, that an object which originally is attended to with effort so often comes after a time to be attended to without effort. To look at the printed words in a story book and to think of '4 and 7 are 11' and the like in doing sums in addition, imply effort in the 7 year old child in school, but none in the practiced reader and accountant.

Getting rid of the feeling of effort is due to getting rid of irrelevant impulses or ideas which need checking or inhibition, and to the strengthening of the relevant impulses or ideas by their repetition and resulting satisfaction. Just as a person could free life as a whole from the feeling of effort, if the tendencies to do every thing that he had to do were made a hundred times as strong and the tendencies to do everything that he must not do were reduced ninety-nine per cent. in strength; so in a single process of life like reading, effort vanishes in proportion as the tendencies to do what must be done in reading (*e.g.*, to move the eyes to a point on the line) are strengthened and the tendencies to do what must not be done (*e.g.*, to move the eyes away from the point before the words are perceived) are weakened. There is no mysterious law that effort decreases with repetition. It does not except in so far as the need for inhibition decreases.

Neglect.—Selecting one thing implies the disregard of other things. For one feature of a mental state to be focal, others must be kept in the margin. Attention has, as its corollary or negative aspect, neglect.[1] The same

[1] The term inhibition is the one commonly used for this process

process is, from the point of view of the thing selected, attention, and, from that of the thing disregarded, neglect. The account just given is then as applicable to the latter as to the former. Tendencies to neglect, like tendencies to attend, are partly inborn and partly acquired. The laws of their acquisition are the same; discomfort being the rejecting and dissociating force as satisfaction is the emphasizing and associating force.

Neglect may be intrinsic or derived, according as the object is in itself unattractive or repellent, or has grafted upon it the unattractiveness or repulsiveness of its mental associates. Neglect may be with or without a feeling of strain or effort.

§ 60. *Satisfaction and Discomfort*

Two facts, resulting satisfaction and resulting discomfort, have been constantly invoked as causes of changes in the life of thought and action. The reader is acquainted with these facts in his own experience but certain knowledge about their presence and causation needs statement here. To explain fully why any human being thinks and feels and acts as he does, it is necessary to know what circumstances will give him the feelings of satisfaction and of discomfort. Having learned that connections productive of satisfaction are selected for survival and that connections productive of discomfort are eliminated, the final step is to learn what sort of result is satisfying.

of disregard or neglect. The word inhibition is however used also to mean the prevention of *any* tendency, of tendencies to move, to perceive, to associate ideas and the like as well as the prevention of tendencies to attend to an object. It is best to avoid ambiguity by using *rejection* or *neglect* to refer to the negative aspect of attention and keeping *inhibition* for the more general fact of prevention.

Original nature decides this in part. Man is so constituted by nature that certain stimuli produce feelings of satisfaction and others discomfort. Sweet tastes, rhythmical sounds, movements after rest, relaxation of the muscles after fatigue, the moderate action of the senses of vision, hearing and smell, are thus satisfying to well nigh everyone. The free exercise of instinctive tendencies to take, hold, play, sleep, run, fondle and the like, is an almost equally important source of satisfaction. Sensory pains from blows, cuts, burns, diseases and the like; certain sensations and emotions such as hunger, thirst, fatigue, fear, anxiety; restraint from the exercise of instinctive tendencies, as by capture, confinement or the obstruction of movement, are for the same reason uncomfortable. Let us call these two classes of feelings, *Original Satisfiers* and *Original Troublers.*

Original nature alone is obviously insufficient to account for all likes and dislikes; for they differ much with different individuals, change much with age and alter quickly with training. Whether any given result shall be satisfying or uncomfortable depends in part upon what it has been associated with. The rule is that, other things being equal, any feeling will be satisfying which has been associated with original satisfiers, and that any feeling will be uncomfortable which has been associated with original troublers. Thus 'to have the bottle' becomes a satisfactory result to the baby, being suffused with the feeling originally felt only with the result 'food in mouth.' After the satisfyingness has been acquired from connection with an original satisfier, it can spread further. Later 'to see the bottle being brought' and later still 'to be told "You shall have your milk,"' acquire in turn this aura of satisfyingness. The discomfort of the blow spreads to the sight of the uplifted hand, and from there to the sound of the spoken threat. No matter how barren of instinctive pleasurableness a condition may be, it may become the most cherished and satisfying of feelings. 'I am doing God's will,' 'I am serving the state,' and 'I am hunting the truth,' have ruled men's lives in spite of their lack of intrinsic satisfaction.

The general laws of instinct and of association thus account for the satisfying and uncomfortable qualities of different feelings as well as for the connections amongst stimuli, mental states and movements. How the satisfaction following upon a connection strengthens it, and how the discomfort following upon a connection weakens it, must be left unanswered questions. Neither psychology nor physiology has yet anything much better than a guess to offer to this, the most fundamental question of the mental life of man and of the animal kingdom as a whole. All that can be said is that the original satisfiers are as a rule events useful for the survival of the species and the original troublers are as a rule events disadvantageous to the survival of the species; consequently any means by which the former could reinforce the connections causing them and the latter weaken the connections causing them would, when evolved, be maintained by natural selection. Perhaps their respective influences on the blood supply constitute such a means.

§ 61. *Conclusion of Part III*

Complex as is a human life, it is at bottom explainable by a few principles. The presence of original tendencies to connections and of satisfaction and discomfort as qualities of certain feelings, the power of satisfaction to strengthen the connections producing it and of discomfort to weaken those producing it, the natural influence of frequency, recency and intensity on connections:—these are the ultimate laws of dynamic psychology. Of these the only one unexplained by the general laws of living beings is the power of satisfaction and discomfort.

The development of a human mental life may be likened to that of the animal kingdom as a whole. The present animal kingdom is the result of the existence in the past of many variations, the elimination of those which did not fit the environment so as to survive, and the persistence of the others through heredity. The eliminating agent in this case is death. Any man's intellect and character are the results of the existence in his past of many connections, the elimination of those which did not fit their environment so as to bring satisfaction, and the persistence of the others through the law of association. The eliminating agent in this case is dissatisfaction and the environment is not the physical world alone but also the greater universe of passions and ideals, of wrong and right, of falsehood and truth.

It is often said that there is and can be no science of human nature, that it is impossible to do more than make shrewd guesses as the poets, story-writers and proverb-makers do. The progress of psychology is, however, gradually proving the assertion false. Even in the elementary and untechnical account of psychology presented in these few pages, there is given enough evidence to justify the faith that human life can be the object of systematic and verified knowledge. Nor are the facts of psychology so chaotic and fragmentary as is generally supposed. Although yet far from the perfection of full explanation by a few general laws which is being reached in the case of physical facts, they are nevertheless being more and more reduced to order and summarized under simple laws. In Part I the rich variety of human thought and feeling was shown to be after all divisible into three natural groups; first, feelings of direct experience; second, reproductions of direct experience; and third, feelings meaning or referring to direct experience. In Part II the tremendously complex physical basis of mental life, the nervous system, was shown to be essentially the sum of the connections between sensitive areas of the body and motor organs, the same bodily organ, the neurone, being always the connecting agent. In Part III it has been shown that in great measure the intellects and characters of men are explainable by a single law, and that in the case of certain facts psychology possesses the final warrant of a science, the power to predict the future.

CHAPTER XXI

Conclusion: The Relations of Psychology

§ 62. *The Science of Psychology as a Whole*

In this book only the more elementary and fundamental facts and laws of mental life have been presented. A complete account of the science of psychology would require many volumes. We have studied only the more general facts of ordinary human mental life, but psychology deals also with the details of sensations, the associations of ideas and the like, with the facts of abnormal and diseased minds and with the mental processes of animals. I have, as a rule, described only those facts which may be appreciated by simple observations and reflection, but psychology uses also intricate analysis, elaborate experiments, exact measurements and wide comparisons. The subject matter of psychology covers a wide range of facts, and these are studied by many different methods.

Such a book as this can, of course, be but the slightest beginning of a study of psychology,—of the thoughts and feelings of men, their relation to the nervous system and the human actions which they arouse and guide. The field of the science is so wide, and the methods of studying it so various that any one small book can present only the most general principles and offer only the simplest kind of an introduction to psychology as a whole. During the year 1903 alone there were published over two thousand books and articles on psychology or allied topics, written by recognized scientific workers. These included studies of the psychology of children as well as of adults; studies of the insane, of the feeble-minded and of animals as well as of ordinary human beings; studies of the growth and decay of mind as well as analysis of its normal conditions; studies of the deeper realities behind human lives as well as of mental facts taken at their face value. The psychologists who wrote them used in some cases observation and reflection, in other cases comparison, experiment and measurements. In many cases all these methods were employed. The subject ranged from *The Psychology of Advertising* to *The Psychology of Religion*, from *Habit Formation in the Crawfish* to the *Aesthetics of Unequal Division.*

The Subject Matter of Psychology.—The chief divisions of psychology and the subject matter dealt with by each are:

General Psychology: The ordinary mental life of human beings.

Individual Psychology: The nature and amount of the mental differences which are found among human beings.

Abnormal Psychology: Exceptional and unhealthy mental traits.

Child Psychology: The mental life of children.

The *growth* of mental life in the individual and in the race is often regarded as a special division of psychology and called Genetic Psychology.

Animal Psychology: The mental life and ways of learning of the lower animals.

Physiological Psychology: The relations between mental life and conditions of the body, especially of the nervous system. The division of psychology dealing with the relation of stimulus to sensation is called Psychophysics.

Social Psychology: Those aspects of mental life which are connected with the influence of human beings on one another and the action of human beings in groups.

Educational Psychology: Those aspects of mental life which are connected with the production of changes in human beings, especially by consciously directed human influences.

Philosophical Psychology: The fundamental realities behind the facts of mental life. The place of mental life in the universe as a whole.

The Methods of Psychology.—The chief methods of studying mental facts and the names commonly given to them are:

Observation: Mental facts are noticed (1) directly in oneself by introspection, or (2) indirectly in others by studying their behavior and their statements about their mental lives.

Analysis: Complex mental facts are broken up into their elements. The composition of mental states is studied.

Experiment: Mental facts are noticed under special conditions arranged for the purpose.

Measurement: Quantitative estimates of mental facts and their relationships are made.

Comparison: Any one group of mental facts is studied in the light of others. Human mental life is studied in connection with animal mental life. Adult minds are compared with the minds of children; normal mental conditions with abnormal, etc.

Reflection: All methods imply the thoughtful, logical consideration of facts.

Any one of the kinds of subject matter may be studied by several methods. For instance, Child Psychology may be studied by all the methods except by direct introspective observation. It could be so studied if there were children who were also psychological students. Each method is, however, in the present state of the science, more appropriate to some kinds of subject matter than to others. Thus animal psychology is very often comparative; philosophical psychology is rarely aided by experiments or measurements; individual pschology is much more frequently quantitative than is social psychology. The tendency of the present time is to rely less on mere observation and analysis and more upon carefully planned experiments conducted with quantitative precision.

§ 63. *The Relations of Psychology to Other Sciences*

Psychology is related to other sciences both as a dependent and as a contributor. It needs the results of physiology to explain the action of the nervous system which is the basis of mental life as we know it. It supplies or should supply the fundamental principles upon which sociology, economics, history, anthropology, linguistics and the other sciences dealing with human thought and action should be based.

The connection between psychology and physiology has been illustrated so often in this book as to need no further comment. Everywhere we have to seek for the physiological basis of mental facts and connections. Through physiology, psychology makes connection with anatomy, physics and chemistry. The structure of the body must be known if we are to understand the action of the sense organs, central nervous system and muscles. The nature of the physical forces must be known if we are to understand the ways in which the sense organs are stimulated by outside events. With some of the physical sciences, such as geology, astronomy, physical geography, paleontology, botany and mineralogy, psychology has only the most remote relations.

With the non-physical sciences, the connections should naturally be closer. The story of human life as told by anthropology and history; the picture of man's dealings with man given by sociology; the analysis which economics makes of human action in the production, distribution and consumption of wealth; the record of the processes of human thought which is stored up in languages,—all these should furnish material for the student of human thought, feeling and action. On the other hand, the facts and laws of psychology,—its account of why human beings think and feel and act as they do,—should provide the general basis for the interpretation and explanation of the great events studied by history, the complex activities of civilized society, the motives that control the action of labor and capital, and the causes to which linguistic inventions and modifications are due. Theoretically, history, sociology, economics, linguistics and the other 'humanities' or sciences of human affairs are all varieties of psychology. But in fact the connections have not been close. These sciences have not attained sufficient insight into general principles or sufficient precision in the knowledge of details to offer psychology very many valuable contributions. And psychology, for the same reasons and also because the greater part of its endeavors so far have been confined to the one problem of the way we come to feel the world of things,—to perceive space, color, form, movement, weight and the like,—has not been a necessity to students of these sciences. On the whole, psychology has at present more to gain than give. But in the future psychology will undoubtedly assume the relation to the other sciences of human affairs which physics now holds to geology, meteorology, astronomy and the like; it will become the fundamental science in the mental world.

§ 64. *The Relations of Psychology to the Arts*

The sciences state facts and laws; the arts give rules for practical procedure. Science seeks to know the world; the arts, to control it. Each art is or should be dependent upon some science or sciences for its general principles. Thus the rules of the art of architecture should be derived from the laws of mechanics, aesthetics, etc.; the practice of medicine and surgery should be founded in the sciences of physiology, pathology, bacteriology, anatomy, etc.; the art of steel-making depends upon the facts of chemistry and metallurgy.

If there were a complete science of psychology,—if the laws of human nature were fully known,—all the arts concerned with human thought, feeling and action would be based upon it. The orator and actor would seek from psychology knowledge of the laws governing the feelings of an audience; the man of business would ask from psychology an account of the motives which influence men in buying and selling; the teacher would derive his methods from a consideration of the psychological laws of learning; the statesman would study psychology to find the probable effect on a population of a certain law or policy; the manufacturer would obtain the advice of a psychological expert concerning the conditions under which his employees would work most intelligently and efficiently.

Psychology is not sufficiently advanced as yet to give the man engaged in the control of human forces much more useful knowledge than he can obtain by direct observation of his own special problems and common sense inferences from what he sees in daily life. And the only practical sphere in which there has yet been any important relation between the science of psychology and the arts of control over mental life is that of education. In this case the value of the science has been perhaps exaggerated. The art of teaching has been improved by being based upon the science of psychology, but not so much as one might hope.

As the science progresses, it will more and more provide with useful rules all the arts that aim to influence men, and will more and more be recognized as a part of the equipment of the teacher, business man, clergyman, employer, statesman or writer. Even now there are signs of a rapidly growing recognition of its importance by practical men.

Psychology and Education.—Education was mentioned as the one art which has been commonly supposed to rest upon a foundation of psychology. The supposition has a far better warrant now than it had fifty or even ten years ago.

Besides the general recommendations concerning the best ways to get boys and girls to study, to notice, attend to, understand, remember and apply knowledge, to form habits and develop capacities, which spring out of the facts of general psychology, there are three lines of special psychological knowledge which are influencing the practical work of education. (1) The psychology of childhood has acquired facts concerning instinctive tendencies, the gradual maturing of capacities, the tendencies useful and harmful in children's habits of observing, associating and reasoning, the actual kinds and amounts of knowledge which they may be expected to possess at different ages and under different conditions, their likes and dislikes, the relation of their mental to their physical well being and the like. You will hardly find a book or address on the art of teaching before 1890, which pays any attention to the fact of instinctive tendencies and you will hardly find one after 1900 which does not. The knowledge of these facts is altering the treatment of children in homes as well as in schools. (2) The results of researches in dynamic psychology, mostly quantitative, into the nature and amount of individual differences, the relative shares of original nature and experience in the formation of human intellect and character, the relationships between various factors in education and certain traits of mind, and other allied topics, are being studied by the men and women who plan educational systems, construct the programs of studies for the schools and select the methods of teaching to be followed,—who, that is, administer the affairs of education. For instance, the old practice of trying to get everyone in a class to the same level of achievement is fast vanishing as a result of increasing knowledge of individual differences. (3) The detailed studies of special topics, such as the time taken to perceive objects, or the nature of eye-movements, or the course of fatigue, or the relation of motor skill to intellectual capacity, frequently provide some fact or theory upon which those who have charge of school systems or classes of scholars base changes in their practice. For instance, manual training, though introduced into the schools largely because of the belief that in some subtle way the acquisition of bodily skill improved the intellectual powers, is coming year by year, as later studies show this relationship between bodily skill and intellect to be not at all close, to base its claims rather upon the value of the knowledge of physical things, the appreciation of industry and art, the actual skill and the interest in constructive activity which it produces.

§ 65. *The Relations of Psychology to the Personal Conduct of Life*

Knowledge of psychology should make one better able to control his own mental life. Man is more nearly master of his own intellect and character than of anything else in nature. The mind is readily influenced, the nervous system being the most modifiable of all the bodily organs, and one has a power over himself that he has over no other mind. 'Psychologist, improve thyself' is an even more just command than 'Physician, heal thyself.'

The application of psychological knowledge to the work of self-improvement has important limitations, however. The first is due to the same fact that limits its application to the arts of controlling others,—the incompleteness of the science: we do not know enough about psychology to give us self-knowledge and self-control.

In the second place, making the most of one's own intellect and character depends largely upon the knowledge of one's own individual psychology, of the mental characteristics peculiar to oneself, of one's special variations from the common human type. But this knowledge the study of general psychology does not supply; it must be gained by direct observation. In the third place, the habit of taking an impartial, purely scientific view of oneself is rare. To see ourselves as others see us, or as a scientific observer would see us—who of us even tries to do that?

Even with the limitations of the inadequacy of psychology, the indispensability of direct observation of individual make-up, and the rarity of a scientific attitude toward oneself, psychology can minister to the art of self-improvement. Although this book presents but the outlines of the science, it should teach a number of lessons in the conduct of life. A brief mention of some of these may indicate what the student could expect from further knowledge of psychology.

It is a natural tendency, when disturbed by any unpleasant fact, to do one thing after another blindly in the hope of getting rid of or altering the fact. This holds of mental as well as bodily life. If we find that we are not very well liked by some companion, we do this or that to please him in a hit or miss fashion; if we grow irritable during the day, we try to work it off in a fit of scolding or we go out doors for a tramp or we do nothing; if we become discouraged and pessimistic, we resort to prayer or to drink or to a change of air as our habits may be, from no rational idea of what is the matter with us or what is its best remedy. Now every step in psychological study teaches us that for everything in mental life there is a reason, that what anyone thinks or feels or does at any time is the result of causes, and that these are to at least some extent knowable. When in mental difficulty, do not worry or aimlessly try this or that, but *seek the reason,* is the plain teaching of psychology. The advice is worth following. The cause will not always be found; when it is found, to avoid it or to find a remedy for its action will in some cases be impossible. But there will be very many cases where an intelligent search for the reason of a mental fact will soon disclose both it and the means of preventing it.

Too often the energy of life is wasted in sickly thought or unproductive emotion. Life is wrecked morally for anyone who is content with fine thoughts and fine feelings. Psychology, in teaching us that the function of mental life is to arouse and guide action, warns us against the errors of the sentimentalist and emotional enthusiast. The lessons of church and of school are unfortunately often insufficient, and even misleading, here. To feel love toward God and righteousness, to thrill with admiration for the heroes of history and fiction, to say fine things about truth and duty—these are too often accepted as virtues in and of themselves. Psychology teaches us that they are worthy only in so far as they are expressed in worthy conduct,—that, as mere feelings, they may even be vices because they may encourage the habit of feeling satisfied with being a wolf in action with a sheep's clothing of sentiment. This is a sound lesson. Not only the hateful Pecksniffs and the charming Sentimental Tommys, but every one of us, needs it. You think and feel so as to do, and what you do—that and that alone you will really be.

It is a common fallacy in human conduct to try to do a thing merely because someone else has done it with success. Jones made a fortune by speculating in stocks. Why not I? Miss Smith went on the stage and is a great actress. Why not I? The reason why is that you are not Jones or Miss Smith. The fallacy is the neglect of differences in capacity. To know our powers and our limitations is the first step in using them wisely. Many of our failures are due to forgetfulness of our limitations; many of our missed opportunities are due to forgetfulness of our powers. We spoil a first rate artisan to make an inferior lawyer. She who might be happy and useful as a wife and mother becomes a dissatisfied and inefficient teacher. Psychology teaches us to take stock of our mental equipment and to wisely dispose our forces in the attack on life's problems, to seek carefully for the lines of least resistance.

Perhaps the most important of all the practical lessons of psychology is furnished by the general law of the modification of the mind by every thought and feeling and act of a man's life. Common experience teaches us in a vague and partial way that what we are at any time depends upon what we have been and done in the past; but life is so complex and the causes of the growth of intellect and character are so hidden that unless we have studied mental life scientifically we are almost sure to make two errors,—to suppose (1) that much in our lives is due to chance and (2) that by an act of will we can at any time blot out the past and begin again. Psychology proves and reinforces the practical conclusion of the wise men of all ages that every thought and act of life counts, that we build the ladder by which we climb, that nothing happens by chance. Though we seem to forget what we learn, each mental acquisition really leaves its mark and makes future judgments more sagacious; a few indulgences in some useless or bad habit are of small consequence but they are of some consequence; nothing of good or evil is ever lost; we may forget and forgive, but the neurones never forget or forgive. Balzac somewhere says that if a young man is upright and honorable till he is twenty-five he can never become thoroughly vicious. It is certain that every worthy deed represents a modification of the neurones of which nothing can ever rob us. Every event of a man's mental life is written indelibly in the brain's archives, to be counted for or against him, not at some far off judgment day, but in every future step of his mental career. We must learn then that no intellectual or moral response is without importance and dignity. The influence of each one lasts as long as life; the little things prepare for the great; no effort for truth and right is ever a waste; no error should ever be without regret. We must learn to have full confidence that we shall think wisely and act nobly in face of the great problems and decisions, if we do the measure of our duty by the common day's work of thought and action. Our only responsibility toward the unknown is to do our best by the known. He who is faithful in a very little is given authority over ten cities.

Man not only creates his own future by the responses he makes from moment to moment; he also creates in some measure his own present by his power to select what features of his surroundings shall influence him. The psychology of attention should teach us that in some degree we can literally make the world. We can avoid the pain and distress and cherish the joy and hope. It is our choice whether the world shall be sordid and mean or inspiring and noble,—shall be ugly or beautiful, encouraging or disheartening. There is no place in nature so repellent as to possess no feature which attention might select to enjoy; nor is there any place so lovely as not to make dissatisfied one who should focus a fault-finding mind on some one of its details. We are as truly and perhaps as much rulers as victims of circumstances. As saints burning at the stake have felt only the joy of worship, so we may refine away the dross from life simply by not attending to it. To banish great physical pain or impressive misfortune is perhaps too much to expect of ordinary mortals, but surely there is no excuse for any student of psychology who does not keep his stream of attentive thought turned away from minor discomforts and mishaps, petty irrelevancies and idle regrets.

One of our chief practical problems is to conduct life so that we may think and act rightly with as little effort or strain as possible. Effort or strain is what makes work unpleasant in the doing and destructive of mental health, and the worker a trial to all his friends and associates. It is our duty to them and to ourselves to work easily, without fatigue and irritation. Psychology teaches us that mental activity is in itself pleasant, that to think is more enjoyable than to be empty-minded, that the effort and strain of thought and action are not concerned with the actual thinking and doing, but with *not* thinking and *not* doing,—with inhibiting irrelevant ideas and undesirable impulses. The effort involved in reasoning we found, in Chapter XVII, to be due to the irruption into our stream of thought of ideas which did not fit our purposes and so needed to be promptly ruled out of the mind's court; the effort involved in voluntary action we found, in Chapter XVIII, to be due to the rise of impulses which conscience or wisdom could not approve and which the will must promptly squelch. The effort of being industrious is the effort not to heed the calls of idle pleasures. We become weary, worn and peevish because of what we do *not* do.

Psychology offers us help in two ways. In the first place tension and effort may be lessened by so arranging circumstances that undesirable ideas and impulses requiring inhibition will seldom appear. The school-boy who cannot do his lessons in the midst of the family circle often works successfully if given a study room for himself. Men for whom the moral life was a bitter and wearying struggle have found peace and rest in the monastery. Every intelligent worker soon learns that discretion is often the better part of valor, that to avoid temptation is often wiser than to resist it. Psychology also teaches us to distinguish between those impulses which should be overcome by never letting them come to the front, and those which should be faced and conquered outright. The rule is simple. Any undesirable impulses which must be often met sooner or later need to be absolutely inhibited: any which are transitory, infrequent and unnecessary in life may best be avoided. It is the error of the weak individual to always either yield or avoid; it is the error of the strong mind to make needless victories, expensive in their tax on the power of inhibition; it is the error of all of us to fight useless battles,—useless either because, being weak, we are sure to be beaten or because, though strong, we gain victory at too great a cost.

In the second place much of the need for voluntary inhibition is due to a misleading notion taught to many of us in school that the harder work we make of any mental task, the better we shall do it. 'I must now make a tremendous effort at concentration, bend all my energies to the work, gird up my loins for an intense fight,' we say, with the expectation that the amount of effort that we expend will decide the amount of work that we get done. Nothing could be more perverse. Other things being equal, the more easily we work, the more we shall accomplish. The success of mental work is measured by the amount done and its quality, not by the feelings we have when doing it. The most efficient workers make the least display of effort; and the best men and women morally are those who do what is right with the least moral struggle. The mental attitude toward intellectual work should be to think, not of our efforts, but of the problem in hand. We should do right with as little trouble to ourselves or anyone else as may be.

As a last illustration of the applications of psychology to the practical control of life, we may take the outcome of the general fact that our feelings of things and of personal conditions are due to conditions of the body. Common sense has by the present day come to agree that a headache is more likely to come from overeating or eye strain than from anxiety or disappointed love, and that the temper and peevishness of children are caused by improper food rather than by the sin of Adam. Psychology extends the lesson through the entire realm of sensation and the sensory emotions. Of course, improving one's health is not the only way to improve one's temper, but it is the easiest. Correcting eye defects is not the only way to increase the quantity of one's mental work, but it is one of the most profitable. A sagacious school principal who realized the effect of the physical functions on intellect and disposition remarked that he looked especially for teachers who had strong 'insides.' Certainly one of the best means of preserving intellectual vigor and emotional balance is to maintain healthy 'insides.'

These samples may serve to show that psychology has a real bearing upon mental hygiene. At the present time its recommendations are necessarily somewhat vague, but with every advance in the science of mental facts we may rightly expect a corresponding advance in the art of controlling them.

Concerning the general position of psychology amongst other sciences and in relation to the arts, the facts given in this chapter emphasize the incorrectness of the common notion of psychology as a study apart from the recognized sciences and devoid of meaning for the practical affairs of life. On the contrary psychology is intimately connected with the biological and social sciences and is likely in the future to become one of the most useful of them to the practical man.

References

A. Stout, *Manual,* 14-32.
Titchener, *Outline,* §§ 5-6.
Angell, *Psychology,* pp. 3-10.
B. Ebbinghaus, *Grundzüge,* § 6.
James, *Principles,* VII.

TOPICS FOR SPECIAL STUDY

The topics and references given below are chosen to meet the needs of students in their first year of psychological work, who wish or need to make an intensive study of several topics. Those marked (A) may conveniently be studied by all students and even before any text-book is completed. Those marked (B) should in most cases be studied only by interested and capable students and after the text-book is nearly or quite completed.

The aim in the selection of references has been not only to name books and articles by thoroughly qualified experts, but also to name only those which are not too advanced for college students, which can be readily obtained by the ordinary college or normal school class, and which exist in an English text. Books known to be out of print, such as Galton's '*Inquiries into Human Faculty*,' are for this reason rejected; and articles in periodicals which the student would be unable to buy and of which a single copy or none would be found in his institution's library, are used very sparingly. It is unfortunately true that not one in fifty amongst college and normal school students of psychology can read a technical book in a foreign language. All the books referred to may well be bought for the library of any institution which offers instruction in psychology.

In some cases the reference is not to pages to be read but to sets of experiments to be done. Such cases are marked *Experimental*.

(A) 1. The Nervous System. *The Growth of the Brain*, by H. H. Donaldson, or *The Anatomy of the Central Nervous System*, etc., by L. Edinger (translation).

(A) 2. Sensations. Chapters I-VII of *An Introduction to Physiological Psychology*, by T. Ziehen (translation), or *The Analysis of Sensations*, by E. Mach (translation).

(A) 3. The Sense Organs. *The Physiology of the Senses,* by J. G. M'Kendrick and W. Snodgrass.

(A) 4. The Experimental Study of Connections of Impression. Chapters V and VI of *Analytical Psychology,* by L. Witmer. *Experimental.*

(A) 5. Vision. *Sight,* by J. Le Conte.

(A) 6. Color Vision. *The Colour Sense,* by Grant Allen, or *Colour Blindness and Colour Perception,* by F. W. Edridge-Green.

(B) 7. Hearing. *L'Audition,* by P. Bonnier.

(A) 8. The Experimental Study of Perception. Chapters I and IV of *Analytical Psychology,* by L. Witmer. *Experimental.*

(B) 9. The Perception of Space. Chapter XX of *The Principles of Psychology,* by W. James, or *Studies in Auditory and Visual Space-Perception,* by A. H. Pierce.

(A) 10. Illusions. *Illusions,* by J. Sully.

(A) 11. Hallucinations. *Hallucinations and Illusions,* by E. Parish (translation).

(A) 12 Apperception. *Apperception,* by K. Lange (translation).

(B) 13. Apperception. *The Reading of Words; A Study in Apperception* (in the American Journal of Psychology, 1897, VIII, 315-393), by W. B. Pillsbury and *The Apperception of the Spoken Sentence* (in the American Journal of Psychology, 1900, XII, 80-130), by W. C. Bagley.

(A) 14. Attention. *The Psychology of Attention,* by T. Ribot.

(B) 15. Imagery. *Mental Imagery* (Monograph Supplement No. 7 of the Psychological Review), by W. Lay, or *An Essay on the Creative Imagination,* by T. Ribot (translation).

(A) 16. Memory. *Memory,* by F. W. Colgrove, or *La mémoire,* by J. J. Van Biervliet.

(B) 17. The Association of Ideas. *Association* (Monograph Supplement No. 2 of the Psychological Review), by M. W. Calkins, or *L'association des idées,* by E. Claparède.

(B) 18. Reasoning. *The Psychology of Reasoning,* by A. Binet (translation).

(A) 19. The Physiological Basis of the Emotions. Chapter XXV of *The Principles of Psychology,* by W. James and *Les émotions* or *Ueber Gemüthsbewegungen,* by C. Lange (translations from the Danish).

(A) 20. The Expression of the Emotions. *The Expression of the Emotions,* by C. Darwin.

(B) 21. Fear. *Fear,* by A. Mosso (translation) and *A Study of Fears* (in the American Journal of Psychology, 1897, VIII, 147-249), by G. S. Hall.

(B) 22. Anger. *A Study of Anger* (in the American Journal of Psychology, 1899, X, 516-591), by G. S. Hall.

(B) 23. Joy. *The Emotion of Joy* (Monograph Supplement No. 9, of the Psychological Review), by G. V. N. Dearborn.

(A) 24. The Instincts of Animals. *Habit and Instinct,* by C. L. Morgan.

(A) 25. The Instincts of Man. Chapter XXIV of *The Principles of Psychology,* by W. James and Chapters III-XIII of *The Fundamentals of Child Study,* by E. A. Kirkpatrick.

(B) 26. Movement. *Le mouvement,* by R. S. Woodworth.

(A) 27. Suggestion and Hypnotism. Chapter XXVI of *The Principles of Psychology,* by W. James and one of the following: *Hypnotism,* by A. Moll (translation); *Hypnotism,* by J. M. Bramwell; *The Psychology of Suggestion,* by B. Sidis.

(B) 28. Diseases of the Will. *Diseases of the Will,* by T. A. Ribot (translation) and *Les obsessions et les impulsions,* by E. Régis and A. Pitres.

(B) 29. The Self. Chapter X of *The Principles of Psychology,* by W. James and Chapter VII of Book IV of *A Manual of Psychology,* by G. F. Stout.

(B) 30. Physical and Mental Fatigue. *Fatigue,* by A. Mosso (translation), or *La fatigue intellectuelle,* by A. Binet and V. Henri.

(A) 31. Dreams. Chapter IV of *Sleep,* by M. de Manacéine (translation) and *Les rêves,* by P. Tissié.

(B) 32. The Acquisition of Skill. *Studies in the Psychology of the Telegraphic Language* (in the Psychological Review, 1897, IV, 27-53 and 1899, VI, 346-375), by W. L. Bryan and N. Harter, or *The Practice Curve*

(Monograph Supplement No. 19 of the Psychological Review), by J. H. Bair, or *Studies in the Psychology and Physiology of Learning* (in the American Journal of Psychology, 1903, XIV, 201-251), by E. J. Swift.

(A) 33. The Inheritance of Mental Capacities. *Hereditary Genius,* by F. Galton, or *Mental and Moral Heredity in Royalty,* by F. A. Woods.

(B) 34. Sex Differences in Mental Traits. Chapters VI-VIII, XII-XVI and XVIII of *Man and Woman,* by H. Ellis, and *Mental Traits of Sex,* by H. B. Thompson.

(A) 35. Experimental Psychology. *Experimental Psychology and Culture,* by G. M. Stratton, or *The New Psychology,* by E. W. Scripture, or *Analytical Psychology,* by L. Witmer.

(A) 36. The Psychology of Infancy. *The Mind of the Child,* by T. W. Preyer (translation), or *First Steps in Mental Growth,* by D. R. Major.

(A) 37. The Psychology of Childhood. *Studies of Childhood,* by J. Sully, or *The Fundamentals of Child Study,* by E. A. Kirkpatrick, or *Notes on Child Study,* by E. L. Thorndike.

(A) 38. The Mental Life of Animals. *Animal Behavior,* by C. L. Morgan, or *Animal Intelligence* (Monograph Supplement No. 8 of the Psychological Review), by E. L. Thorndike.

(B) 39. The Psychology of Primitive Man. *The Basis of Social Relations,* by D. G. Brinton, or *Primitive Culture,* by E. B. Tylor.

(A) 40. The Psychology of Races. *The Psychology of Peoples,* by G. Le Bon (translation), or *La psychologie du peuple français,* by A. Fouillée, or *The Russian People* (in *The Expansion of Russia,* by A. N. Rambard), by Novikov Yakov.

(A) 41. The Psychology of Insanity. *The Pathology of Mind,* by H. Maudsley, or *Sanity and Insanity,* by C. Mercier.

(A) 42. The Psychology of Intellectual Superiority. *English Men of Science,* by F. Galton and *A Study of British Genius,* by H. Ellis.

(B) 43. The Psychology of the Feeble-minded. *The Mental Affections of Children,* by W. W. Ireland, or *The Psychology of Mentally Deficient Children,* by N. Norsworthy or *Mental Defectives,* by M. W. Barr.

(A) 44. The Psychology of the Mob. *The Crowd,* by G. Le Bon (translation), or *L'opinion et la foule,* by G. Tarde.

(A) 45. The Psychology of the Criminal. *The Criminal,* by H. Ellis.

(A) 46. The Psychology of the Deaf-Blind. *The Story of My Life,* by Helen Keller, or *Laura Bridgman,* by M. H. Elliott and F. H. Hall and the article on *Laura Bridgman* in *Aspects of German Culture,* by G. S. Hall.

(B) 47. The Psychology of the Weather. *The Weather,* by E. G. Dexter.

(A) 48. The Psychology of Play. *The Play of Animals* and *The Play of Man,* both by K. Groos (translations).

(A) 49. The Psychology of Religion. *The Varieties of Religious Experience,* by W. James, or *The Psychology of Religion,* by E. D. Starbuck, or *The Spiritual Life* and *The Religion of a Mature Mind,* both by G. A. Coe.

(A) 50. The Psychology of the Occult. *Fact and Fable in Psychology,* by J. Jastrow.

(B) 51. The Psychology of Speech. *The Faculty of Speech,* by J. Collins, or *Aphasia,* by F. Bateman.

(B) 52. The Development of Speech. Chapter V of *The Psychology of Childhood,* by F. Tracy, and *Die Entwicklung von Sprachen und Denken beim Kinde,* by W. Ament.

(B) 53. The Psychology of Reading. *On the Psychology and Physiology of Reading* (in the American Journal of Psychology 1900, XI, 283-302 and 1901, XII, 292-312), by E. B. Huey, or *Psychologische Untersuchungen über das Lesen,* by B. Erdmann and R. Dodge, or *The Psychology of Reading,* by W. F. Dearborn.

(B) 54. The Psychology of Spelling. *Spelling in the Elementary School,* by O. P. Cornman.

(B) 55. The Psychology of Arithmetic. *The Psychology of Number,* by J. A. McLellan and J. Dewey.

(B) 56. The Psychology of Writing. *Zur Psychologie des Schreibens,* by W. Preyer.

(A) 57. The Psychology of Advertising. *The Theory of Advertising,* by W. D. Scott, and *On the Psychology of Advertising,* by Harlow Gale (pp. 39-69 of his *Psychological Studies*).

(A) 58. Psychology and Philosophy. *An Introduction to Philosophy,* by F. Paulsen (translation) and Chapters V and VI of *The Principles of Psychology,* by W. James.

(B) 59. Psychology and Philosophy. *Why the Mind Has a Body,* by C. A. Strong, or *The Philosophy of Mind,* by G. T. Ladd.

(B) 60. Psychology and Ethics. *The Psychology of Ethics,* by D. Irons.

(B) 61. Psychology and Aesthetics. *Aesthetic Principles,* by H. R. Marshall.

(B) 62. Psychology and Sociology. *The Psychic Factors of Civilization,* by L. F. Ward, or *The Principles of Sociology,* by F. H. Giddings, or *The Laws of Imitation,* by G. Tarde (translation), or *Etudes de psychologie sociale,* by G. Tarde.

(B) 63. Psychology and Economics. *La psychologie économique,* by G. Tarde.

(A) 64. Psychology and Education. *Talks to Teachers on Psychology,* by W. James, or *Genetic Psychology for Teachers,* by C. H. Judd, or *Herbartian Psychology Applied to Education,* by J. Adams, *or The Principles of Teaching,* by E. L. Thorndike, or *The Psychological Principles of Education,* by H. H. Horne.

Bibliographies of Psychology

The books and articles on psychology which have been written since the beginning of 1894 are carefully indexed in the annual *'Psychological Index'* of the *Psychological Review.* A selected bibliography containing the titles of all important books on psychology is being published as a volume of the *Dictionary of Philosophy and Psychology,* edited by J. M. Baldwin.

Guidance in the selection of reading may be best obtained from the reviews of psychological books found in the leading psychological journals. Those in English are: *Mind: A Quarterly Review of Psychology and Philosophy; The American Journal of Psychology; The Psychological Review; The British Journal of Psychology;* and *The Journal of Philosophy, Psychology and Scientific Methods. Nature* and *Science* also furnish trustworthy guidance.

INDEX

Illustrations

Experiments

Names and Subjects